Structural Energetics in Zero Balancing Bodywork

of related interest

Cupping Therapy for Bodyworkers
A Practical Manual
Ilkay Zihni Chirali
ISBN 978 1 84819 357 4
eISBN 978 0 85701 316 3

BodyMindCORE Work for the Movement Therapist
Leading Clients to CORE Breath and Awareness
Noah Karrasch with Robert White and Elizabeth Buri
ISBN 978 1 84819 338 3
eISBN 978 0 85701 295 1

Zero Balancing
Touching the Energy of Bone
John Hamwee
Foreword by Fritz Smith, MD FCC Ac
Illustrations by Gina Michaels
ISBN 978 1 84819 234 8
eISBN 978 0 85701 182 4

Body Intelligence Meditation
Finding Presence through Embodiment
Ged Sumner
ISBN 978 1 84819 174 7
eISBN 978 0 85701 121 3

Awakening Somatic Intelligence
Understanding, Learning & Practicing the Alexander Technique, Feldenkrais Method & Hatha Yoga
Graeme Lynn
ISBN 978 1 84819 334 5
eISBN 978 0 85701 290 6

Structural Energetics in Zero Balancing Bodywork

● ● ● ●

ALAN HEXT

Foreword by Fritz Frederick Smith, MD

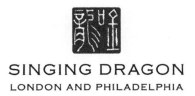

SINGING DRAGON

LONDON AND PHILADELPHIA

First published in 2020
by Singing Dragon
an imprint of Jessica Kingsley Publishers
73 Collier Street
London N1 9BE, UK
and
400 Market Street, Suite 400
Philadelphia, PA 19106, USA

www.singingdragon.com

Library of Congress Cataloging in Publication Data
A CIP catalog record for this book is available from the Library of Congress

British Library Cataloguing in Publication Data
A CIP catalogue record for this book is available from the British Library

ISBN 978 1 84819 375 8
eISBN 978 0 85701 332 3

Printed and bound in Great Britain

This book is dedicated to those discovering, learning, practising and teaching Zero Balancing.

Contents

Foreword

Fritz Frederick Smith, MD, Founder of Zero Balancing

Alan Hext is a senior Zero Balancing practitioner and teacher, a master acupuncturist, and a serious student of Chinese medicine and the Chinese classics. He and I became good friends after first meeting in the mid-1970s and he later became one of three people instrumental in bringing Zero Balancing into the UK. The inception of Zero Balancing actually occurred in England during my first year of acupuncture training at Professor J.R. Worsley's College of Chinese Medicine, Kenilworth, England. I had met J.R. Worsley several months earlier when he presented an acupuncture programme at the Esalen Institute, Big Sur, California. He and I had an instant and deep connection. One evening we were standing on a bluff overlooking the Pacific Ocean when he said to me: 'Fritz, I wish you could see the world the way I do, through the wisdom of the five elements of Chinese medicine.' As I read *Structural Energetics in Zero Balancing Bodywork*, I understood even more deeply the wisdom which J.R. Worsley referred.

In his book Alan views the system of Zero Balancing through the windows of acupuncture, the Chinese classics, Chinese characters and the teachings of J.R. Worsley himself. In describing Zero Balancing and structural energetics, Alan continually references qi energy and the importance of the concept of pairings, fundamentally expressed as yin and yang, the sunny and shady sides of the mountain: 'It needs to be remembered that it is a single mountain and yin and yang are the double aspects of the one.' In Zero Balancing, structure and energy are the fundamental pairing we work with, the underpinnings of the body, understanding that they are a reflection of the 'one'. Alan flushes out amazing new richness, relationships and potentials of Zero Balancing, and presents the reader with a deeper understanding of body/mind therapy. In many places he weaves Zero Balancing so beautifully with the Chinese classics that his book might be regarded as the 'Chinese anthology of Zero Balancing'.

Acknowledgements

I would like to thank all those with whom I have studied and who have attracted me to learn authentic practices. Fritz Smith, MD, the founder of Zero Balancing, has been an inspiration in my journey of discovery. I am forever grateful to him for his generosity as a teacher and for his continuing support and encouragement.

Professor J.R. Worsley opened the door for me to practise acupuncture. He brought the nature and essence of the traditions alive, and proved their value in clinical practice.

Claude Larre and Elisabeth Rochat de la Vallée awakened my heart-mind to the wisdom and inner meaning in the Chinese classics.

I thank my Taiji Quan teacher Master Choy Kam Man and others transmitting Cheng Man Ching's teachings.

Alan Watts originally attracted me to study Oriental culture and practices.

Thanks also to my partner Alice Rogers for her help, to Stephen Dew for his skills with illustrations and to Claire Wilson for inviting me to write, and to all at Singing Dragon for their guidance in the publication of this book.

Disclaimer

The fulcrums and methods in this book are for descriptive illustration. They require formal instruction and training for their proper practice.

No medical claims are being made in this book. The reader should seek appropriate professional care and attention for any specific healthcare needs.

Introduction

If you are reading this in the form of a book, the structure you are holding in your hands has a spine. You have engaged with the book by opening its pages. The spine is acting as a central coordinator and an axis that allows you to access its pages left and right, so that they become available to be read. By reading its contents you have activated potential communication and comprehension. These are key aspects of the book's structural energetics.

The essential structural energetics of a human being are that we are vertebral beings with a central spine. We stand vertically upright on two legs. Our head is elevated so that it rests on the top of our trunk. The two girdles of the shoulders and pelvis connect our trunk with the four limbs of our arms and legs. Our hands and feet have a particular anatomy that has structurally and energetically developed through their interaction with our brains.

What is animating our structure? What is the internal regulation that gives our life integrity and unity? What attracts us to stand upright? Zero Balancing provokes curiosity into a breadth of questions, about, for instance, gravity, consciousness, our body-mind and what it is to be human.

We continue to explore, understand and realise who we are as living human beings. Zero Balancing has a part to play in our personal evolution and understanding what it is to be alive. It is a body-mind practice that invites us to awaken to being consciously human. Zero Balancing has a contribution to make to our development as human beings, beyond its recognisable value in nurturing health and wellbeing.

The appreciation of Zero Balancing is comprehended through direct touch, and the limitations of describing practical work by the written word present obvious difficulties. Comprehension requires interactive hands-on education. I remember from my school days the problems of attempting the task of writing instructions on how to tie a necktie. Describing the practicalities and sensitivities required in Zero Balancing has similar challenges. An intellectual grasp is transcended by non-verbal demonstration that directly reveals what is meant by the art and skill of Zero Balancing.

I am writing this in the year in which Fritz Smith, MD, the founder of Zero Balancing, celebrates his 90th birthday. He is testimony to the power of this remarkable form of bodywork to nurture good health and longevity. He continues to actively teach and explore its potential. His biography and the story of Zero Balancing's development is told in the book *Life in the Bones*, superbly edited by David Lauterstein (2017). Fritz has taught Zero Balancing internationally, inspiring thousands of healthcare practitioners to study and practise the skills he developed. As the creator of Zero Balancing he is naturally honoured as the founder. However, he has been clear that Zero Balancing stands independent of himself as an art and skill that can be taught by anyone trained to teach or who is qualified to practise Zero Balancing.

I first met Fritz when I was living in California in the mid-1970s. At that time this area of the world felt as if it was a place of renaissance, discovery and innovation. I was there exploring the different bodywork approaches that were being developed. This State, on the rim of the Pacific Ocean, geographically faces and is culturally open to the wisdom of the Orient. I visited Fritz in his practice and observed him with clients. He would see them for a relatively short amount of time and practise with ease and focus in what appeared to be a simple manner. His clients would drop into deep relaxation, responding with enjoyment to the quality of his caring touch. They would then arise and re-accustom themselves to standing upright on their own two feet. Their first few steps showed them getting used to feeling being in a new body. Their eyes were alive and shining, as if a light within them had been turned on. Something was happening beyond immediate explanation that I had not come across in other therapies.

I deeply appreciate and have enormous gratitude for Fritz's generosity and teaching. From his welcoming me to observe him in practice in the 1970s as part of my acupuncture studies to his personally Zero Balancing all the participants in early workshops over many years, Fritz has, in turn, been even more generative through giving his permission and enthusiasm for Zero Balancer teachers to establish local Zero Balancing organisations in several different countries. Educationally Fritz has encouraged experienced teachers in their explorations of Zero Balancing, giving his approval to teachers creating their own Zero Balancing skills workshops. He has helped Zero Balancing flower through placing his trust in those he has taught as teachers in their presenting new dimensions of the possibilities and application of Zero Balancing.

Fritz has shared his knowledge and insights freely. He welcomes questions with the openness of one who equally learns from your questions. His teaching has that special quality of informing you, an experience of getting it in your hands through the direct experience of touch. It is as if he had shared a treasured gift, one you will know through its practice and which generates a multiplication of this gift through sharing it with others. The sense of revelatory delight that is realised through hands-on discovery is a frequent experience of the joy of learning Zero Balancing. He has taught a therapy that the student can literally get a handle on in their first workshop, whilst realising it has unfolding development as a skill and therapeutic art as their practice matures.

I recognise in Fritz a true Gentleman who embodies being a gentle-man treating everyone with equality and attention. As a bodyworker he handles people with a gentle power that is unforgettable. You feel deeply touched in a non-invasive way, with a clarity and respect for who you are. It can feel like being sculptured, not in a way of being imposed upon, but like a good sculptor who brings out the inherent nature of the material they are working with. You feel realised and confirmed in your true self, returned to your living form.

In Zero Balancing Fritz has literally incorporated many skills that are implicit in the high-level practice of a wide variety of therapies. The academisation of therapeutic skills in modern education can mean that the inner development of the practitioner can become forgotten, marginalised or boxed into just another module. Through the development of conscious touch, Zero Balancing makes gaining rapport tangible. Zero Balancing is 'working with' compared with 'doing to' the patient, and involves the practitioner in a way that is engaging and rewarding. A series of Zero Balancing sessions have an unfolding nature. It is a transformative process rather than the mere application of mechanical techniques or a systemised sequence.

Fritz has presented Zero Balancing not as a belief system, but as an invitation to explore and discover. Students are encouraged to begin a workshop with a 'blank sheet', open to new possibilities. Whilst there is much in a workshop to excite the mind or stimulate the intellect, the process of learning is directly embodied. You 'get it' in your hands and it jumps you out of those approaches in education that separate theory and practice.

I have studied Zero Balancing since 1983 when I took the first workshop that Fritz taught in England. I have richly enjoyed continued studies, becoming a certified Zero Balancer, and in 1989 qualifying as a Zero Balancing teacher. I have developed and taught workshops such as 'The Roots of Zero Balancing in the Chinese Traditions', 'The Structure of Energy' and 'Elemental Zero Balancing'. I use it regularly in my practice as a bodywork in its own right and alongside traditional acupuncture. It continues to be of enormous value, demonstrating and proving its ability to serve patients. I have personally found myriad benefits in my own wellbeing and development as a healthcare practitioner.

This book also draws on insights from classical Chinese culture as pioneers who explored the field of structural energetics in insightful ways. Their insights are pertinent to our own explorations of Zero Balancing. These can aid cross-cultural comprehension, helping us transcend the limitations in our contemporary understanding. Chinese characters have been included to illustrate understandings and insights that their ancient culture already knew and from which we can learn and benefit. I take responsibility for their translation and interpretation in an endeavour to make mystery accessible and the esoteric tangible.

My hope is that this book, first, attracts people to seek out trained Zero Balancers and receive Zero Balancing sessions. Second, that it interests those attracted to study through attending workshops. A continued exploration and learning is then served best by enrolling in the programme leading to certification as a Zero Balancer. And third, that it contributes to the critical understanding of those who have studied and who practise Zero Balancing. They know through their own experience its benefits to clients as well as to those who practise it.

The therapeutic applications of Zero Balancing are manifold, serving our health and so much more. Zero Balancing invites you on an unfolding path of exploration and reflective learning. Dr Fritz Smith has gifted us a true practice that is beyond belief.

1

What is Zero Balancing?

Zero Balancing is a gentle yet powerful method of balancing body energy with body structure using skilled touch. It was developed by an American osteopathic physician, Fritz Smith, MD. Zero Balancing integrates Western knowledge of our body with Oriental insights into energy, recognising the ways our body heals itself and how we maintain good health.

Practitioners of Zero Balancing are healthcare professionals who have been trained to a recognised level of skill and awarded the title 'certified Zero Balancer'.

A Zero Balancing session lasts between 30 and 40 minutes, during which the client remains fully clothed. The work is performed with the client sitting and then lying comfortably on their back on a Zero Balancing (ZB) table. Zero Balancing uses held stretches and finger pressure with a focus on bones and joints. It takes a person into a place of refreshing relaxation, which can bring about a profound experience of wellbeing and body-felt unity. The touch used in Zero Balancing has a characteristic clarity that is pleasurable to receive.

The gentle but firm touch brings about a return of flexibility, encourages good posture and clears stiffness in a richly restorative way. The sensitivity of touch used in Zero Balancing returns us to ourselves whilst simultaneously opening us to an awareness of a centred presence in the world.

Zero Balancing is very useful when we are becoming overwhelmed by stresses in our lives, which can, in turn, lead to a decline in our vitality and our ability to adapt to change. Contemporary life is increasingly attracting us into a virtual experience, with life being lived at an ever-faster pace. Staying in touch with the actual world and its natural rhythms is an essential reality check that is valuable in maintaining the vital balance which is health.

Zero Balancing is beneficial for a wide range of people and effective in many ways. It is truly a bodywork ideally suited for the lives we live now.

Fritz graduated with a Doctor of Osteopathy degree in 1955 and Medicine in 1961. He later studied Traditional Acupuncture with the renowned UK teacher, Professor J.R. Worsley, who awarded Fritz a Master of Acupuncture degree in the 1970s. Fritz also studied cranial osteopathy with the first generation of Dr William Garner Sutherland's students, learning structural integration with Ida Rolf, and yoga and meditation with Muktananda.

Fritz is the author of *Inner Bridges: A Guide to Energy Movement and Body Structure* (1986) and *The Alchemy of Touch* (2005).

Fritz developed Zero Balancing as a project of excellence during his acupuncture studies and taught it to his fellow students. Its name came from a client's description of her experience of a session: 'I feel I've been brought back to balance, like a return to zero.' Dr Smith has taught Zero Balancing internationally, to thousands of healthcare practitioners.

2

A Description of a Zero Balancing Session for the Client

You may have been attracted by reports of friends or been intrigued by the name and curious that this is something different to, for instance, massage or manipulative therapies. What is Zero Balancing?

I would suggest seeking out a certified Zero Balancer. Keep an open body-mind without expectations, and discover its benefits for yourself. A session will be tailored to your own needs whilst following an approach and sequence common to all who practise it. One of its key identifying characteristics is the quality of its touch and the way you are handled.

The session begins with an initial discussion with the Zero Balancer so they can have a clear idea of your particular needs, health history and any medications being taken.

Zero Balancing is performed with you comfortably lying on your back, fully clothed.

It begins with some initial evaluations with you in a sitting position on the side of the ZB table. The Zero Balancer stands behind you, contacting your back with a clear touch. You feel they meet you with their fingers as if they know where and who you are in your body. The touch has a firm clarity as your ribs are contacted in a rhythm which brings you present in yourself.

The Zero Balancer then takes your arm, moving it in a circular motion, and ending with a gentle rocking movement which seats it in the shoulder joint. They then move to your pelvis, siting their thumbs on your sacrum and asking you to gently rock from side to side, ending with the instruction 'return to centre'.

Other evaluations may be made to understand how you are in any body areas you may have highlighted. A session can be like a tour of your body whereby you discover areas of sensitivity you were unaware of. You become aware of how your body has been aided by how you have exercised or used it, or how it has been affected by stress or injury. It can feel as if you are being introduced to yourself through informed and sensitive touch.

You then lie down on the ZB table on your back. Your head is comfortably placed on a low pillow that is checked for correct height.

A session then usually follows a protocol that addresses the whole body in an ordered sequence. It begins with the lower half of your body and then continues on your upper body, followed by movements that integrate the work, bringing the session to a sense of completion.

The Zero Balancer holds your body at the ankles and introduces a gentle traction that you can feel throughout your body. It is held for a short while and you feel becoming settled in yourself, relaxing on the ZB table.

The Zero Balancer then brings their hands under your pelvis and makes contact with your sacrum, close to where the sacroiliac joint lies. The quality of touch has a firm clarity whilst having a sensitivity. You feel your bones being contacted in a way that is respectful and affirming. The touch invites you to rest in your body, releasing layers of tensions you hadn't realised were there. This is touch you can trust. You relax deeply within yourself. You instinctively know you are in 'good hands'.

Your mid and lower back are evaluated, beginning around the floating ribs and upper lumbar area. You may become aware of tensions you didn't realise you were holding. The Zero Balancer surveys the whole lower back, including the pelvis, feeling the inter-relationships between different areas.

The Zero Balancer may ask you how the level of their touch is for you. It helps in modulating touch so that it accurately works with you effectively. The nature of the touch both meets and engages you, bringing new levels of awareness of your body so you know better who you are in yourself.

A variety of fulcrums (see Chapter 3) are introduced and held for a short time and then released. There is a rhythm and sense of interaction, which is like having a conversation by touch. You feel engaged and held in a way that invites you to participate. The rhythm of touch, gentle holds and stretches, removal, pause and proceeding to another area has an intelligence and completeness to it. The rich layers of interrelationships are being recognised, rather than being handled as bit parts. You begin to sense the wider whole of being one within yourself.

Each leg is carefully lifted and your hip joints are evaluated and fulcrums introduced. The evaluation may bring you into being aware of possible restrictions in, for example, the internal and lateral rotation of one side. The movement is performed with a clear focus, as if you were being shown the nature and mobility of the joint hidden deep in your pelvis.

The fulcrums open up the hip using held stretches and movements that engage and release. They have an acceptable comfort of working within the range of movement you are familiar with. You may feel this way of working with your hip also engages the pelvis and its joints. You can feel the tension in hip movement release as you return to a smoother quality of hip movement you hadn't realised was lost.

The rhythm of evaluation, fulcrums and re-evaluation continues throughout the session. It has an intelligence interaction giving working feedback that is beneficial to you and the Zero Balancer. The Zero Balancer is working with a thorough attention whilst you feel you are able to keep track of and informed of change as a participant. The Zero Balancer then evaluates and Zero Balances your feet.

The Zero Balancer then nestles their hands high on the arch of your foot with a firm, comfortable hold. This is a fulcrum you are aware you could not do to yourself. It also engages your whole leg, building on work already done, so you feel it build on and integrate with the areas of the body already touched.

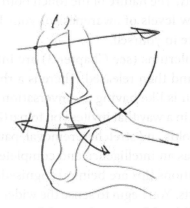

Evaluation of the tarsal joints and foot fulcrum

The work brings a welcome feeling to your feet as they come alive. The pressures of standing on your own two feet or the footwear you've worn in life or the way you've used your feet are all there to be touched and worked with. You may be reminded of the freedom you knew in your feet earlier in your life as layers of tension clear. Your body breathes a welcome sigh of relief.

The Zero Balancer may return to areas previously worked and then gather it all together, introducing a gentle stretch that engages the whole lower half of your body.

They then move to the head of the ZB table, and sit behind you. They may well check in with you, enquiring how you are getting on. This feels a genuine enquiry and does not interrupt your experience of the session. Indeed, it confirms the sense of attention you are receiving, and that you are both working together.

Their hands are brought under your upper back and your ribs are palpated. As with your lower back, it may yield discoveries of places of sensitivity unknown to you.

The upper body is evaluated in its interrelationships, your shoulders' girdle and the movements of your head and neck. The head is respectfully moved through a range of motions, then return-ing to being held with a gentle curved traction. You become aware of your head and neck in relation to the whole of your upper body. It feels so good to be reminded of a central alignment.

The Zero Balancer returns to the ribs. You notice the feeling of bone being touched with well-placed holds at places along the length of the ribs identified in the previous evaluation.

The touch can have a quality of being a 'good ache', one that touches but does not disturb. Fulcrums are held for a short time as if they were welcoming your response. You are aware of a level of deep relaxation, dropping into a place where you are being truly met.

Following a range of work on the whole of your upper back and neck, the Zero Balancer may choose to include an interactive fulcrum holding your head-neck. You are given instructions so you work with them, moving your head whilst they engage it in a gentle hold. When your head is then placed down on the pillow, you may feel the release in the whole area. Your breathing may go into a deeper relaxed rhythm, pause, and then fill your body, taking a full breath.

The Zero Balancer may let you know that they are moving towards completing the session and check in with you as to whether there are any other areas of your body requiring attention.

The session then moves into a series of integrating holds and gently held stretches. These confirm the experience of being centrally aligned.

Your arms may be picked up, engaged with a gentle stretch, and returned to lie on the front of your body. There is a sense of all the whole session being brought to a fulfilling and satisfying completion.

The Zero Balancer may gently squeeze your heels as a non-verbal indicator that the session has arrived at its conclusion. The squeeze and hands removed give a clear ending. You may lie on the ZB table for a short while, taking in the enjoyment of how your body feels, and a relaxed refreshment.

You may be in a place of deep peaceful rest whilst also feeling fully awake. You can feel internally still whilst aware of the rhythms of your body, such as your breath. There can be a sense of quietude, of being in meditation.

Roll carefully onto your side, pause for a moment, and then slowly sit up on the side of the ZB table. Take a moment to feel what it is to sit, feeling the uprightness, before putting both feet down together on the ground. Step down onto both feet as you come off the ZB table.

You may be encouraged to walk in a line in the room, to help integrate the session. This activates your body and aids the assimilation of the Zero Balancing into your whole body.

Clients sometimes report feeling taller, or as if they are floating in their body. Others say how relaxed they feel with a pleasurable freedom that they discover on moving. There may be alterations in your sense of time. The duration of the hands-on work was 30 minutes, but it feels as if time has been suspended and the session lasted much longer. There may be a combination of relaxation, freedom of movement and improved coordination.

On walking outside, the colour of the trees and flowers may appear more vivid and the beauty of the natural world becomes alive.

In my experience as a receiver I was told that, the day after the session, I might feel slight muscle aches, as if I had done more physical work than usual. However, this was not the case. What was most noticeable was, having felt like an early night, I enter into a level of deep restful sleep that has hitherto eluded me, waking the next morning feeling renewed. I actively want to get on with my day, including addressing things I'd been avoiding dealing with.

The Zero Balancer suggested I would benefit from a handful of weekly sessions that would build on the work of the first. Later on, the time between sessions was lengthened, or I saw the Zero Balancer according to my needs or attraction to receive Zero Balancing.

I had a particularly demanding time coming up and returned for more sessions that helped me negotiate my way through a period of life which otherwise I know would have taken its toll on me. I found dealing with people I had previously found difficult or meetings that had been fraught both seemed to go smoother. In fact, what I thought were impossible situations changed, with mutually satisfactory outcomes. I felt more attracted to take care of myself. I am now able to know there are different ways of being in my body that help me being at ease, so tensions affect me less and don't accumulate.

People who come for Zero Balancing sessions report saying, 'I really feel met', 'The touch had just the kind of contact I needed', 'I felt held'. Being handled with a high level of respect was a quality of touch that I could fully trust. It allowed the work to free me and let me drop into a deep place of rest: 'I felt brought back to myself, to who I am'.

There are several good descriptions of Zero Balancing sessions in print that describe individuals' experiences. Several are recorded in detail in Dr Fritz Smith's *The Alchemy of Touch*, or there is a variety of case studies in *Experiencing the Power of Zero Balancing* (Quarry and King 2016), from practitioners in the UK and USA.

3

Learning Zero Balancing

Healthcare practitioners from many disciplines have found enormous value in learning the body-mind therapy of Zero Balancing. It encapsulates in practical ways many high-level skills aspired to in a range of therapeutic approaches. It does so in an embodied way rather than merely knowing them as theoretical ideals.

There are now qualified teachers of Zero Balancing who hold workshops in many different countries such as the UK, USA, Switzerland, Spain, New Zealand and Mexico.

Dr Fritz Smith developed Zero Balancing as a practical bridge between orthodox medicine and alternative, complementary medicine. For therapists who use a physically based approach, it introduces tangible ways of working with the energetics of the body and of reading the resultant changes. For those already working with approaches that involve energy, it teaches ways of contacting the body's structure that can ground their work in a new and effective manner.

Touching the Body's Structure and Energy Simultaneously

Zero Balancing teaches the art and skill of the coordinated handling of body structure and body energy. *Body structure* refers to everything that is in a state of relative stability. *Body energy* covers everything that is in relative movement, ranging from circulation to the subtlest energy flow. A Zero Balancing session encourages the optimal balance between structure and energy to nurture the harmony of wellbeing and good health.

Being Touched at the Level of Our Bones

To be touched with care and attention at this level of our structure is enormously affirming of our core sense of being. This is a distinctively different experience to bodywork approaches that focus on soft tissue. Our skeleton, being made of the densest matter, conducts some of the strongest energetic currents. To be simultaneously touched at the level of our bones and the energy flowing through our form is a specific hallmark of Zero Balancing.

Developing a Working Rapport with the Client

Zero Balancing develops a special relationship between the client and practitioner that nurtures deep levels of instinctive trust. This level of sensitive rapport with each individual involves the client being actively engaged in the session, even though to a superficial observer they may appear to be a passive receiver. This bodywork is one that works *with* the person, rather than merely doing something *to* them. It makes its practice a richly satisfying therapeutic approach for both practitioner and client.

A Vocabulary of Touching Energy

Zero Balancing develops the conscious use of human touch. It distinguishes different qualities of working with energy. Zero Balancing develops a specific tactile sensitivity that maintains clarity between the practitioner and client. It means that the client is able to go through changes in a session without any confusion of identities between themselves and the practitioner. For the Zero Balancer it cultivates the ability to be fully present with the client, attentively serving their needs with clarity, respect and compassion.

Fulcrums and Vectors

The hands-on tools of Zero Balancing are known as *fulcrums* and *vectors*. They provide an orientation around which the client's structure and energy can respond. Being relatively neutral and non-manipulative, they offer the client the opportunity to change and rebalance. This opens up the possibilities of not only structural alignment but also internal transformation, returning a person to themselves.

Deep Relaxation

Zero Balancing encourages a person to access a state of conscious relaxation in which gentle touch can open them to fundamental change. In this state more can be achieved with less effort. Simple, accurately placed fulcrums and vectors engage the client and can lead to beneficial responses well beyond normal expectations.

Evaluation, Balancing and Re-evaluation

The Zero Balancer follows a working method that grounds this bodywork in a rhythm that gives them clear feedback loops. Such tangible observation of how the client is responding is of great value in customising and pacing each session to the needs of the individual. In Zero Balancing, practitioners learn to feel and evaluate the client's structure and energy through simple movements of the client's body joints. Following the work with fulcrums and vectors, the practitioner re-evaluates and thereby stays in hands-on touch with the client, their response and the process of the session.

The Significance of Particular Joints

Within our skeletal structure are several joints that have a minimal range of motion and whose function is related more to the transmission of energetic forces. These joints, such as the sacroiliac joint, are known as foundation joints and are of key importance in

Zero Balancing. When such joints become imbalanced, the body tends to compensate in ways that can have widespread effects that we may not be aware of. The subsequent compensations can impede our functioning and set up unconscious tensions that lead to a reduction in our vitality and disturb our wellbeing.

Working Signs of Internal Change

A person can have a range of involuntary responses during a session that indicate that they are in a 'working state'. The practitioner observes these inner changes that reflect what is happening within the client. Recognising and monitoring these signs informs the Zero Balancer, helping them to serve the particular needs of the individual and guide the pace and rhythm of each session.

Learning a Protocol for a Core Zero Balancing Session

In a core workshop a protocol is learned that provides a clear guide as to how to work effectively with the whole person. These guidelines provide an overall structure for a complete and satisfying 20- to 30-minute session. They are infinitely adaptable to the needs of the individual client.

Altered States of Consciousness

Zero Balancing works with beneficial altered states of consciousness in a session that can assist the client in transcending limitations in a safe and grounded context. Such changes in perceptions are rec- ognised as frequently accompanying healing transformation and awakening to fresh insights.

Opportunities to Study Zero Balancing

Zero Balancing bodywork is taught in various formats. This was originally in a five-day workshop that potentiated its trans- formative experience for those attending. The teaching interweaves presentations of theory with interactive practice. This allows the development of learning with an embodied comprehension, so that practitioners have it in their hands. Practical work is interactive learning guided by feedback from whom practitioners are working with and a Zero Balancing teacher. The process of learning is similar to that seen in disciplines such as Taiji Quan or yoga. Regular practice deepens comprehension and embodiment of the skill.

Ongoing Exploration

Learning Zero Balancing opens practitioners to a journey of discovery that stimulates a natural attraction to developing their skills. The foundations are taught in two core workshops from which it is fully possible to see significant responses and to grasp the fundamental skills. There are a range of further workshops and courses of study that develop comprehension and refine practitioners' Zero Balancing touch, increasing the possibilities of applying it in their practice. Fritz developed workshops such as 'Freely Moveable Joints' and 'Alchemy of Touch' to further the work presented in the core workshops. Other Zero Balancing teachers run approved workshops that provide a particular focus for expanding skills and comprehension. The programme leading to certification as a Zero Balancer is an excellent focus for a practitioner's journey of individual development.

Zero Balancing incorporates inner principles of working which, when used in coordination, activate the practitioner's high-level attention. In an educational context it is a good example of understanding a practical and theoretical skill in which self-reflection is a natural awareness in the process of the practitioner's embodied comprehension. The development of the art and application of Zero Balancing can lead to it becoming a valuable therapy that is a truepractice.

4

Working with the Body's Structure and Energy

Knowing how to touch a person's structure and energy effectively is an essential skill for practitioners to discover in learning Zero Balancing. It is a skill capable of extensive development. As bodyworkers, practitioners are always learning how to modulate their touch to each individual, different areas of their body, and adapting to varying conditions.

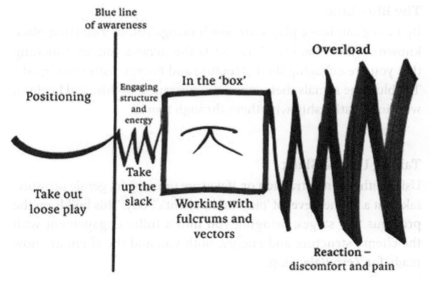

The steps to working with structure and energy

The diagram on the previous page, developed by Dr Fritz Smith, illustrates in a straightforward way the key stages to be aware of in developing awareness and ability to touch. It identifies where a practitioner is in engaging and working with structure and energy, and defines a protocol that can provide accurate feedback.

Positioning

Place yourself in relation to the person and ZB table so you can use your body with ease and effectiveness. This involves becoming conscious of how you use your own structure and energy.

There is a certain amount of free play in the body, often in the musculature, and you need to know how to engage this in the client so that any looseness is taken out. There may be degrees of, for example, hypermobility or lax tone that may become evident from your initial evaluations. This observation will inform the way you handle the client. The curve in the diagram visually represents this beginning stage of 'taking out loose play'.

The Blue Line

By taking out loose play your touch brings you to a starting place known as the 'blue line'. This alerts the person you are touching that you are engaging their structure and energy with your hands. The blue line signals their conscious awareness of this, and begins a working relationship with them through touch.

Taking Up the Slack

Using either gentle traction or, if you are pressing in, gentle pressure, take out a further level of 'play' in the client's body. This builds on the previous two stages, bringing you into a fuller engagement with the client's structure and energy. Both you and the client are now ready for Zero Balancing.

In the 'Box'

Having clearly built the previous stages, any additional movement on your part takes you into the area in which Zero Balancing is performed. You can now introduce fulcrums or vectors of Zero Balancing, building them in different planes as required. The box is an area in which you can Zero Balance the client's structure and energy effectively. Observe any signs of working response that may confirm your working engagement. You may always directly enquire by asking them how a certain fulcrum is feeling.

The box is an area in which you have activated the person's structure and energy with your own structure and energy. Your prior evaluations will help you know their body and how much play and slack you need to engage to arrive in the working box area.

Then, introduce fulcrums and vectors, holding them in place, allowing them to do their work. Re-evaluate, feeling and seeing what has happened. The character of this working interaction in Zero Balancing is like a non-verbal conversation you have with the person through touch. If this is effective and they beneficially respond, it can be like a meaningful conversation. They 'hear' and 'read' your touch and Zero Balancing, and it is understood as meaningful communication.

Overload

Please be aware that if you go beyond the box you potentially stray into areas of touching the person that may feel uncomfortable or even painful for them; they then react rather than respond. You may be aware of this by the feel of your touch, and they may well also let you know.

Releasing

When your fulcrum is completed you need to know how to come out of what you have built. Do this by reversing the stages you have introduced, and then disconnect by taking your hands off the person and returning their body back onto the ZB table.

The body's structure and energy can be activated and engaged in several ways. In practices such as yoga it can happen by positioning the body in alignment, then stretching the body along with relaxation of the breath. In Taiji Quan, for example, you stand, positioning yourself in alignment, relax down into your body taking up the slack, and then move smoothly through the form, with movements originating from the lower centre.

It is possible to 'go through the motions' of both practices and only partially or superficially work your body's structure and energy. Then one day, for instance, in practising Taiji, having learnt the form, you relax into it, move, and it all comes alive and meaningful. Something has been activated. Taiji starts doing you. You go through the form with a new ease, feeling its benefits in your body and mind that you hadn't been aware of before. You embody Taiji.

The value and importance of learning Zero Balancing by working with fellow practitioners is that they are able to feed you back as to the level of your touch through their informed awareness.

Zero Balancing touches body structure and body energy, holding them as one. Structure can be recognised as everything that is comparatively stable in relation to everything that is in comparative movement.

The structure in our bodies that Zero Balancing particularly touches is our bones, the most relatively stable tissue in our body. Body energy embraces the range of everything in relative motion such as our circulation and warmth, our breath, tone and conductivity, vibrational rhythms, the movements of qi energy and subtler manifestations of life, nonetheless tangible to touch.

This working distinction and skill can be found in a multiplicity of other situations. For example, you are currently engaged in reading. The pages of the book and these words are relatively stable whilst your eyes adjust their focal range and move over the sentences in a systematic movement. Together they are then interpreted by giving meaning.

When you write using a pencil, the paper is relatively stable whilst you engage it and move the pencil at just the right level of pressure to create meaningful writing.

A true art and skill is learning how to touch the living body and how to touch a human being in a meaningful, respectful and accurate way. Developing this skill is one of continuing cultivation as you learn to adapt to handling different people, in different conditions and different areas of the body.

Ida Rolf, who developed Structural Integration, said, 'It is not necessary to straighten the Grand Canyon, you just have to make sure water flows through it.' Activating clear communication in the body's structure and energy and harmonising their relationship is the skill of Zero Balancing.

This awareness and these skills are of wider importance beyond bodywork. It is possible, for example, to examine the body's structure independent of its energy or functioning.

An X-ray or MRI scan can reveal our interior structure that is not perceptible by other investigations. A scan can appear 'normal' and yet the person is aware of degrees of suffering that are not evident from just the structure. Another person's scan can reveal considerable structural deviation from the norm and yet they are unaware of any discomfort. What is being missed?

Some investigative procedures in a medical examination require being performed with care and the permission and trust of the patient. If training in anatomy has only been of the body's structure from dissection or texts, there may be missing sensitivities when examining a living human being.

5

Distinguishing Ways of Touching Structure and Energy

Developing a Vocabulary of Touch

Once you are able to touch structure and energy and hold them simultaneously, it is essential to be able to distinguish the variety of ways in which this can happen, and to know these with discernment. Zero Balancing distinguishes several ways in order to be able to recognise these, and chooses to work with touching at the interface.

How do you use your structure and energy to be in contact with another's structure and energy? What can happen in this relationship? It is valuable to be informed of the nature of how these may be used, both in the therapeutic context as well as having ramifications in wider relationships in life.

These distinct ways are presented in order to educate and be able to identify them as part of developing conscious touch. They are not presented pejoratively, but are part of an ability to know a vocabulary of touch.

Definitions

Interface

Touching a person at interface is defined as 'I know where I end and you begin, and I begin and you end'. Interface is the touch of choice in Zero Balancing. The attention is at the fingertips, where you are in touch with another person. You are both at the place where you are meeting each other.

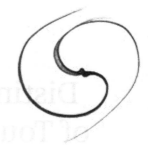

Interface

Interface allows a clear distinction as to who you are individually, whilst knowing the place where you meet. The boundary is not a separation. You can both be present and know whom you are engaged with in a working relationship. The neutrality of this relationship can, in turn, develop a positive energy that catalyses transformation. Through working with interface touch in your interaction, the transformation is one that the other person can know and own as their own.

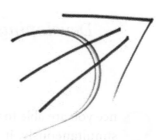

Streaming

Streaming

Streaming is the extending of the practitioner's energy into another person, to intentionally influence them.

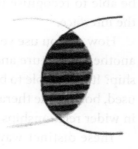

Blending

Blending

Blending is a deliberate lessening of specificity of the place where the practitioner and client meet each other,

Ways of touching structure and energy

allowing both energies to merge. It can lead to a blurring of individuality as energies flow into each other.

Channelling

The practitioner opens themselves up in order to act as a conduit for an energy that is greater than themselves, becoming a channel for this force (not included in the accompanying illustrations).

Let us now look at the characteristics of these different ways of working.

Characteristics

Interface

Touching at bone level whilst simultaneously sensing the energy of life at the practitioner's fingertips helps the clarity of contact and in turn the clarity of the interrelationship. Involving both the practitioner's structure and energy and the client's structure and energy at the interface means both know who they are and also where they both are. It activates their interactive participation in the Zero Balancing in ways that may occur beneath their conscious awareness. This allows them to actively respond, which is empowering whilst bringing clarity of distinction as to who each of them are.

Touching at the interface is a highly respectful level of touch. It meets the person in ways that are both sensitively engaging and non-imposing or developing a divisive barrier. This lessens any confusion of identities. It lessens the possibility of unnecessary influences affecting the practitioner from the client, whether they be colds, emotions, projections or transference.

Touching at the interface conserves the practitioner's energy whilst maintaining their attention and involvement. This can refresh them as well as serve the client.

To bring attention to where the practitioner is working and being at the interface, both practitioner and client become actively present. Both are at the meeting in ways that make Zero Balancing become a bodywork meditation.

Being at the interface is important where fulcrums and vectors offer the opportunity of transformation. The practitioner sets up the conditions whereby balancing can occur, offering an invitation to changes that are real and lasting.

Streaming

Practitioners may have been trained to direct their energy into the other person as part of their practice. It may also be used instinctively, such as by a parent towards a child or loved one when they are suffering distress. Warm, caring energy is instinctively streamed into them. An acupuncturist may needle a significant point away from an area needing help, and through the needle stream into the person the energy of the element along the pathway to influence a distal place – for example, a point on the foot may be used that has a response on the patient's upper body or head. Streaming requires the practitioner to have a stronger energy than the client, and for the client to be in receptive need.

The practitioner may possess a natural tendency to want to give of their energy and be of service to others. However, giving out all the time can lead to the practitioner burning out. It can even provoke resentment from the client when there is no agreed consent, or their expectation is unfulfilled and they are unappreciative. It can lead to a tendency in the therapeutic relationship whereby the client becomes dependent on the influence of the practitioner to actively fix them. They may come to believe or project on the practitioner that they need the practitioner in order to get better.

Blending

When the practitioner blends with the client they deliberately weaken any sense of boundary between them both. Each enters into each other's field. The practitioner may use blending in order to gain a sense of what is happening within the client, and find information empathetically as a non-verbal insight. The practitioner and client may experience a resonant oneness that has the feel of a cosy kind of caring trust and common understanding. However, this may create levels of dependency or lead to difficulties in clarity or separating from a blurred confusion as to who both are.

Channelling

Channelling allows energy to flow through you for the benefit of others. You may, for example, be channelling the lineage of your traditions or drawing on the authority of a founder, the power of a teacher or a belief for whom you are acting as a conduit for this force. This requires the practitioner (channeller) to be a pure instrument, clear in themselves and tuned to the universal. Otherwise the force can potentially be affected by the practitioner's own history or level, and may distort the purity of the force being channelled. The practitioner may also begin to believe that it is they who are the source of energy they are drawing on, rather than simply being the conduit for a universal energy beyond their personality.

Knowing the range of differing ways of touching structure and energy can be a revelation to practitioners. It can give them an insight into ways of relating they may have been instructed in or they may be personal unconscious tendencies. The practitioner's education or history means that they may also have favoured or deliberately developed certain ways of touching people that they use ubiquitously and are unconscious of.

This vocabulary of touch allows the practitioner to work consciously with a wider appreciation of their possible consequences and interaction.

6

Signs of Response and Change

I n studying Zero Balancing there are several practical and theoretical aspects that are essential to learn in order to practise:

- Where to touch

- Ways of evaluating

- How to touch

- Working with fulcrums and vectors

- Ways of monitoring response

How does a Zero Balancer know from observing the client in a session that they are touching structure and energy in a significant way?

There are a range of responses, known collectively as the 'working signs', which indicate a person's structure and energy is being activated beneficially. They are perceptible signals that happen involuntarily in the client, and indicate that the client is in a 'working state' during a session.

These indicators have been gathered by careful observation and are not unique to Zero Balancing. This can be a valuable observation for practitioners in a wide range of different therapies. Being sensitive to observing these 'signals' can be of great value as part of appreciating feedback from their therapy and in the process of working with individual clients.

When Dr Fritz Smith was studying and observing J.R. Worsley practise acupuncture, he was particularly struck by the ways J.R. Worsley would know when a person had responded well, and also by how he was able to recognise that any treatment was 'complete'. These signs are involuntary and subliminal and a natural part of the client's working responses. They may be unaware that they are happening. These signs can be observed repeatedly in a wide variety of people. They therefore have the truth of being an objective observation. Whilst some people may only show a few such signs, it is important to recognise that any apparent absence of working signs does not mean that beneficial change is not happening.

The working signs indicate that the person is in a working state of Zero Balancing. This is described as a period of internal rearrangement, reorganisation and integration which can happen following a shift of balance or vibration.

The work of Zero Balancing is functioning beyond a mechanical cause and effect so the signs may arise out of the relationship of working with specific fulcrums and vectors. They are also part of a wider response of working together in a productive relationship. They are the external signs of the activation of internal energetic change.

The working signs can also be a useful indicator of the sensitivity and responsiveness of the individual client. They can act as a beneficial guide to the pacing of a session, so the client is served by the Zero Balancing without being overloaded.

Dr Fritz Smith has written extensively in his book *Inner Bridges* of these signs (1986), so I simply review them here as they are such a valuable observation.

There are key signs that give the clearest signals of the client's response and are the more important indicators. The major working signs are observable in the eyes, breath patterns and the quality of vitality in their vocal expression.

It should be noted that clients are not given any specific instruction as to keeping their eyes open or closed. During Zero Balancing their eyes may begin to glaze over or appear to be at rest. The eyes, which are usually looking out at the world around us, are now in between external and internal vision. The client's eyes may naturally close. The eyelids may then go into involuntary fluttering, usually considered as reflecting beneficial changes in brain wave activity.

Another involuntary response is variations in the person's breathing, which it is valuable to be attentive to. The cycles of the client's breathing can change from going into temporary shallow breathing or apparent suspension of breath to then being followed by a full breath, which can be like a release. The rhythm of working with fulcrums and changes in breath is a fascinating study just in itself.

There may be a minimum of verbal conversation between the practitioner and client in a session. The practitioner, however, may often check in with the client. This may happen when the practitioner moves to work on the upper body and enquires as to how the client is getting on. The practitioner pays attention to the quality of the client's voice as the indicator, rather than only the words they speak. This gives an insight into their internal state. The practitioner may vary the pace and nature of their touch accordingly, as well as change the duration of the session.

Other working signs are none the less important and may occur as a frequent part of a session.

It can be common to hear a gurgling or rumbling in the client's digestive tract, known as borborygmus. I normally let the client know that this is a positive sign, indicating a beneficial response, which reassures them.

A sense of inner peace can often be seen on the client's face during a session. Such serenity reflects deep levels of relaxation throughout their whole body. They may have a beatific appearance, as if they had returned to being at home within themselves.

Any bodyworker is familiar with changes in their client's tissues as a tangible indication of working response. The process of evaluation, fulcrums and re-evaluation reveals whether such change occurs. Musculature and fascia may become more pliable, reflecting distinct changes of state. As an analogy, I am reminded of kneading wheat dough in bread making, and the way the proteins of the gluten change character when they are worked, becoming 'elastic'.

If there are times during a session when energy becomes unlocked or shifts, then the client's body may go through involuntary movements as it adjusts to new configurations and fields of inter-connection.

There are other signs that can exhibit themselves across our senses, such as changes in colour, expression and odour. These are the external indicators of internal change.

Such a 'vocabulary' of observation of energetic responses complements the development of the perceptions of ways of touching known as the vocabulary of touch in Zero Balancing. They are both important sensitivities to cultivate in a Zero Balancer.

7

An Anatomy of the Energy Body

One of the most perceptive bodies of knowledge of our structural energetic anatomy is that investigated by the Chinese. It fulfils the double function of an energy anatomy – to connect the individual to the greater whole and to enable them to function as an autonomous system. This is a comprehensive structural energetic anatomy that incorporates the individual and the universal.

Whilst this structural energetic anatomy is accessible within our muscles and fascia, it is important to understand it as functioning within the structure of the whole body. The power of its animation is there in the depths of our form, from our bones to the surface of our skin, and includes our organs and senses.

The wealth of knowledge of what is known in China as the Jing Luo (經 絡), or sometimes Jing Mai, incorporates a meaning of vital circulation. This knowledge has a richness which complements that of the structure of the body explored thoroughly over recent centuries in the West. The anatomy of our structure, observed through careful dissection, is present in a dead cadaver. The question is: what is the structure and energy that brings this form alive?

The classical Chinese insight into our form through the Jing Luo is of a living fabric with an integral organisation of warp and weft. The *jing* are the vertical threads from above to below and below to above, with their complement, the *luo*, providing a complementary horizontal interconnection. This is intrinsic to its material life and unity.

As our tendency to consider the anatomy of our structural energetic body is limited to only our structure, we can miss many essential perceptions in this Chinese knowledge. A major one is in the name of the character *jing* (經). The etymology of the character is of a flow of water under the ground, which may not be immediately perceptible on the surface. This flow would be of interest to the geomancer looking at the flows within the land to auspiciously site a building. The character is qualified by the inclusion of the silk radical that gathers this into a wider thread of meaning relevant to the geography of the living landscape of our body.

The warp of our vertical structural energetic functioning unifies above to below and below to above. This connects us with the forces of heaven and earth, which are maintaining us in their complementary fields, bringing us into being and giving us a sense of being in harmony in nature living on this planet.

The character *jing* (經) may be familiar from another context of its use. It is the same one used for *I Jing*, the *Classic of Changes*, and is frequently used to identify writing that is classic. Why? A work is honoured as a classic because although it was written in a particular time, place and culture, its wisdom has living relevance beyond those parameters. The structural content of the book and the energy of its expression are so interwoven and exemplary that it lives as a work in its own right.

The knowledge of the Jing Luo was documented in *Nei Jing*, the *Inner Classic*, over 2000 years ago. The value of its insights is validated by it still being used therapeutically over the whole world over 2000 years later.

This wider meaning of *jing* is important as it is implicit in the way in which a living form maintains its natural order. The meaning is one of maintaining regulation and an ordering of true alignment, which is the inner balance of being in vital relationship.

In the wider life of our societies we know that one way of maintaining order is by legislation. This is an external attempt to try and regulate. The Jing Luo are internal, inbuilt, and therefore integral to our structural energetic regulation on multiple levels.

The more recent translation of *jing* as channel, whilst giving a sense of a structure through which something may flow, conveys none of this inherent regulation. It has the possibility of reducing the true meaning of Jing Luo to a structure of corporeal plumbing!

The choice of the word 'meridian' to describe the Jing Luo pathways was made by a pioneering French diplomat and medic, George Soulié de Morant. As an aside, his archive is now in Yunnan University in China, in a museum I have visited dedicated to the transmission of Chinese medicine to the West. The word meridian is used for the lines of longitude of circumpolar global inter-connection between north to south, by which we regulate clock time and location.

Now, when the first astronauts went into orbit, none of them expected to see the lines of longitude and latitude on earth from space. It has always amused me that when people dissect the structure of the human body they find nothing, saying, 'We never found any meridians or points', and regard this as proof that they don't exist.

The Chinese character *xue* (穴), used for what we know as a 'point', reveals why. Its meaning is of a hollow under the surface. In the wider world it is a cave. A cave is a place where the earth is missing, giving access to its interior. It is a space with a location within the form of the earth. So a point is a hollow, a void, like a breathing space, something genuinely not there.

Other Chinese characters used for what we call points include ones of gates or doorways, places that can open and close through which we gain access in both directions.

One Chinese character for points is *shu* (俞), frequently seen in the point names of the pathway that runs vertically down the back, parallel to the spine. *Shu* contains images of a chariot or boat, with the meaning of something that can travel far. It is emblematic of the nature of points that whilst they have a specific location and will affect their local area, the response will also travel a long way. 'Touch locally and think globally' is very true. When the energy is contacted within the structural energetic body, you are in touch with the whole.

Many acupuncture points lie in the flexures of joints or in the seams of muscles where the breaths of our structural energetic body are being articulated.

When 'points' are recognised as openings and places of reception and communication, they can be properly understood. The emptiness is not a negative but allows essential articulation and storage.

The couple of form and void is a vital perception in the Chinese mind and essential to anyone trying to understand and handle the structure and energy of the body. What is not there is essential for our functioning and might answer questions about life's vitality:

> *Thirty spokes converge upon a single hub;*
> *It is the hole in the centre that the use of the cart hinges.*
> *We make a vessel from a lump of clay;*
> *It is the empty space within the vessel that makes it useful.*
> *We make doors and windows for a room;*
> *But it is the empty spaces which make the room liveable.*
> *Therefore whilst what is there has benefits, it is what is not there*
>   *that allows it to function.*
>
> (Daodejing, *Chapter 11*)

This chapter, from the classic the *Daodejing*, illuminates the essential importance of space/void. It is also displays an inner structure similar to the way the Jing Luo is seen interconnecting heaven, earth and man.

The circle of a wheel is emblematic of the orbits in heaven, clay the substance of the earth, and windows and doors as a metaphor for the upper sense organs in a human being.

The Jing Luo describes the larger picture of a human being, well ordered and balanced in a self-regulating balance. From above to below, below to above, side to side, back and front, interior and surface, all in mutual intercommunication.

Our vertical posture of standing upright is exemplified in a quality of qi energy called Zheng Qi (正 氣). This is translated as upright qi, good health, which is regular and correct for balanced alignment. The norm is for our life and form to be upright. The meaning of *zheng* (正) is of an implicit rectification that occurs when the interconnections between the qi of heaven and earth maintain our natural balance in relation to any influences that might disturb it. When our lives and health are going as they should be, adapting to the changes of the world, and we are fulfilling our destiny, that is, *zheng*, true health is as it should normally be.

In most Western displays of structural anatomy the commonly displayed position is standing with arms beside the body. To properly comprehend the structural energetics of the Jing Luo anatomy, the body is standing with the arms raised and relaxed, held above the shoulders. This brings into alignment the vital interconnection of the pathways within us in relation to heaven and earth. This placement reveals the vertical movement through the length of the whole body of pairings that involve both hands and feet.

8

The Opening Half
Moon Vector

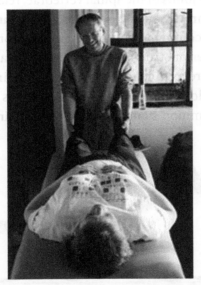

The half moon vector by Dr Fritz Smith

A Zero Balancing opens and closes with a half moon vector, which is also used during sessions to assist integration. Its apparent simplicity conceals its potential power. It is an ideal example to take to explore the dimensions of what is happening in Zero Balancing.

In this half moon vector the Zero Balancer holds the client's ankles in a comfortable nestle, then raises their legs slightly. Engaging the structure and energy of the body, the loose play is taken out and the slack taken up with the introduction of curved traction combined with a degree of dorsiflexion of the client's ankles. This is held with a constancy for several seconds, and the legs and feet are then gently returned to the ZB table.

The client relaxes into themselves and feels at rest on the supportive surface of the ZB table. Working signs may appear such as a release in their breathing as they accept the invitation to settle into refreshing relaxation. They may feel a sense of arriving home, becoming present in their whole body. The half moon vector often engages not only their legs and hips but can also be felt throughout their trunk and up into their head.

The curved traction opens up breathing spaces between the semi-foundation joints of the spinal vertebrae, relaxing tensions and uniting a flow throughout the sections of the curves of the client's spine. This may continue up into the head and brain. The whole of the hidden posterior structure of the legs, back and head becomes connected. The relaxed lengthening is an opening that in combination with the dorsiflexion at the ankles grounds the person within themselves, a common signature of Zero Balancing.

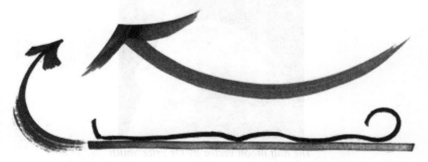

The half moon vector with dorsiflexion of the ankles

In the supine position the spine is not being required to hold us upright, so it can enjoy this communication from below to above and above to below. A sensitive person may also become aware of a pulsation in the front of their body, with the mantramic rhythm of the heart beat complementing the spine, uniting the inner circuit at this central core of the trunk.

When a client arises from a session, stands up and takes a few steps, there is often an experience of being well connected through the heels and feet with the earth. This agile rooting of heels with the ground is complemented by feeling the head floating on top of the spine. The balanced integrity within the body is combined with an awareness that the client is a living connection between earth and heaven.

The activation of central awareness has been referred to as the 'universal flow' through our structure and energy. It is valuable to recall the paired functions of our energetic anatomy – to enable an individual to function as an autonomous system whilst also connecting them with the greater whole.

A small amount of focused activity by the Zero Balancer can result in a response that can be surprisingly disproportionate to the apparent effort. Something is happening within our structural energetics that can appear astonishing, beyond our everyday expectations of cause and effect.

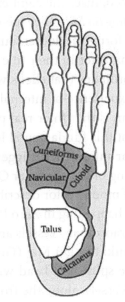

Overhead view of the foot and tarsal bones

Initially Zero Balancing in the UK was described as structural acupressure, recognising both the way it involved the structure at a skeletal level and the meridian pathways as an important understanding of our energy anatomy. Structural acupressure also distinguished Zero Balancing with its bone level contact from other bodywork approaches that use the pathways and points but focus on the soft tissue of the fascia. This half moon vector engages the bladder meridian, the longest pathway in the body, running from the eyes down the entire back and legs to the feet. It can benefit the whole spine without touching it directly. Observing how much of the body registers the half moon vector can indicate areas of held tension.

The 12 meridian pathways follow the vertical length of our bodies relating to heaven and earth, whilst also having an integrity flowing throughout as a unified circuit. Any influence that activates the flow through their length will enliven their verticality whilst also uniting front with back, side with side and interior with surface. This gives an integral interconnectivity of the warp and weft of our living fabric.

Chinese medicine recognises the eight extraordinary vessels, the Chinese name being Qi Jing Ba Mai. They pre-exist the 12 meridians at a level of functioning that forms the deeper foundations of our structure and energy. The first character in their title, Qi, has the meaning of something out of the ordinary that elicits wonder and amazement. My observations and experience of internal Oriental practices such as Qigong or Taiji Quan is that their real power is activated when their practice engages at this fundamental level. Movements that to an observer may appear minor then trigger something that is well expressed by the meaning of the character Qi, marvellous, out of the ordinary. I take the half moon vector described above as an example to explore what may be happening in Zero Balancing.

Two of the eight extraordinary vessels are located on the vertical central lines of the trunk: the Du Mai (Governing or Overseeing Vessel), connecting the spine and head with its complement, the Ren Mai (Conception Vessel), along the front of the body and face.

With its engagement of the whole body through the ankles, the half moon vector can activate another pairing of these primary vessels known as the Qiao Mai (Heel Vessels). These pairings unite our heels directly with our heads, eyes and brain. The Yin and Yang Qiao Mai are often coupled with Ren Mai and Du Mai in recognition of their relationship.

Formatively the extraordinary vessels are fundamental in our formative foetal development, and are essential during the primary stages of childhood development. Young children explore crawling before standing upright on their own two feet. Their heel vessels and core central vessels including the spine are essential to their support and development. They learn how to coordinate becoming an erect human being with their feet on the earth and their head close to heaven.

Standing upright requires distributing our weight through our heels and feet with the rest of the body in vertical alignment. The feet and heels are constantly adapting to different surfaces. The character *qiao* (蹻) is well translated as heel, containing the radical for heel in the Chinese language with the wider meaning of an agile stance that has presence.

The tibia and fibula articulate with the talus as a freely moveable joint, whilst the talus articulating with the calcaneus is a foundation joint. Unlike a freely moveable joint, movement between the talus and calcaneus is beneath our voluntary control, so we are less conscious of their relationship.

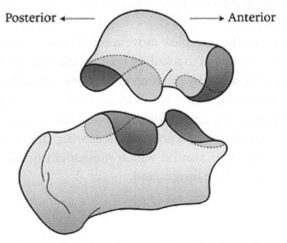

A disarticulated lateral view of the talo-calcaneal joint

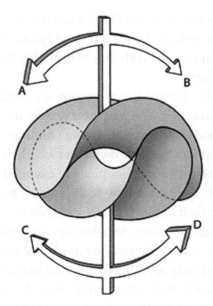

Diagrammatic view of the talo-calcaneal joint

Dorsiflexion of the ankle combines freely moveable and foundation joint actions. The talo-calcaneal articulation is a perfect example of the hidden structural energetic power that is a key aspect of this half moon vector. Each step we take as our heels touch the ground and we shift our weight to walk engages the freely moveable ankle and the talo-calcaneal foundation joint. These are critical to maintain our upright balance.

The nature of the complex movements between the talus and calcaneus can be likened to a sailing boat on the sea. The boat stays afloat on the sea's waves by pitching and rolling, allowing optimum adaptation. When our body is in balanced alignment the vertical forces go through this joint whilst involving the rest of the foot as it distributes the forces of each step. Knowing the centre of this articulation as an axis around which movement occurs is a vital awareness we often take for granted.

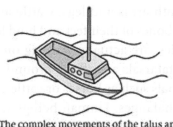

The complex movements of the talus and
calcaneus can be likened to the movements
of a sailing boat on the water

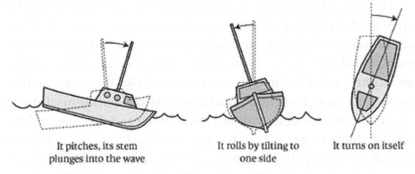

It pitches, its stem   It rolls by tilting to   It turns on itself
plunges into the wave   one side

Movements in the talo-calcaneal joint, like a boat on the sea

Our opposable thumbs of our hands are often cited as the aspect of our anatomy that in combination with brain development is key to making us uniquely human. The talo-calcaneal joints in our heels are perhaps less well recognised but essential to our development as *homo erectus*, the vertical biped. Interestingly, both joints share anatomical similarities in their rich range of possible movements. Both the trapezo-metacarpal joint of the thumb and the talo-calcaneal joint share saddle-shaped articulations of complementary form. They are both known as hetero-kinetic joints, or 'universal joints'. Mechanically this is defined as a joint with two axes perpendicular to each other and comprising two forks that can rotate one to the other at any angle, allowing a multiplicity of movements.

Many mammals are able to stand up almost immediately after being born, as can be seen in quadrupedal four-legged cattle and sheep. A human being, however, only learns to stand upright at the end of their first year, having gone through the developmental stages of crawling using both arms and legs. Cattle and sheep stand on different parts of the bones of their feet and hind legs. Cats and dogs, known as digitigrades, are actually walking on their toes, so that their tarsals and metatarsals are off the ground, giving them extra height. Hooved animals such as horses or cattle elevate even higher, standing on their phalanges. Human beings walk maintaining a different sense of balance with two heels on the ground, a key part of being human.

The two extraordinary vessels of the Yin and Yang Qiao Mai are paired medially and laterally and are rooted in the heel. Their activation and interplay are fundamental in our upright development and stance in the world. Their pathways and influence have an intimate relationship with our brain and also the eyes. Another important aspect of their functioning is the harmonisation of circadian rhythms of activity and rest, waking and sleeping, and the related ability of our eyes to be open or closed. In Zero Balancing one of the frequently observed working signs of this half moon vector is the involuntary fluttering of the client's eyelids. The client's heels are reconnecting the whole of their bodies with their head's brain, and particularly the opening and closing of their eyes. They are awake but at rest; they are neither looking outside nor inside, and have returned to a profound reconnective remembering within themselves.

The Chinese classical text *Nan Jing*, in Chapter 28, describes the two Qiao pathways as 'originating within the centre of the heel' and then manifesting as Yin Qiao and Yang Qiao arising from the medial and lateral sides of the ankle. The two key acupuncture points of the Qiao Mai are located either side of the ankle, just below the central base of the medial and lateral malleoli. They have a relationship with the talus and calcaneus and this joint. Their alternative names are Yin Jiao and Yang Jiao, and they function as the opening 'master points' for both Qiao Mai vessels. In acupuncture anatomy they are medially Kidney 6 (Illuminated Sea) and laterally Bladder 62 (Extended Vessel). It should be noted that in Zero Balancing this half moon vector can be amplified with the addition of a gentle squeeze into the bones of the ankle.

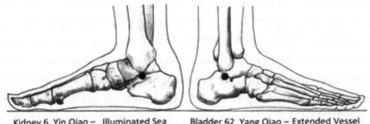

Kidney 6 Yin Qiao – Illuminated Sea   Bladder 62 Yang Qiao – Extended Vessel

Medial and lateral views of the foot with points of the Yin and Yang Qiao Mai

In the name of Bladder 62 (Extended Vessel) – Shen Mai (申 脈), the *shen* has the meaning of stretching out and can also mean being at ease and relaxed. The antonym of this character is *qu* (屈), with the meaning to curl or bend. In this half moon vector a double message is being introduced into the body-mind. The stretch of the curved traction engaging the whole body is conjoined with the curling dorsiflexion at the ankles.

The description of both Qiao Mai is of complementary pathways rising from ankle to head, connecting heel with head and brain. They both unite at a key point beside the eyes, Bladder 1 (Eyes Bright) – Jing Ming. The name reflects not only the brilliance of the eyes but also alludes to the illumination of the mind. We stand upon the Earth with a secure but agile stance, stepping with upright awareness, being consciously awake. One recognised function of the Qiao Mai is to retune a person to harmonious circadian rhythms, particularly the cycles of sleep and wakefulness.

The curved traction of the half moon vector engages the person, offering an invitation to deeply relax and drop into themselves. The level of traction has to be just right for this to engage and activate. Too strong a traction may be felt as an imposition to which they react rather than respond. Too little traction may insufficiently engage them. Just enough brings about a coherent integrity. It is possible to 'separate' the body's structure and energy whereby a person may expand beyond their form, even going outside of or 'leaving' their body. Whilst a sense of release can be useful, such disassociation is not what is happening in Zero Balancing. The correct degree of dorsiflexion of the ankles is essential to anchor someone who may tend to an over-expansive separation of their structure and energy.

I highlight this insight into the extraordinary vessels anatomy and functioning as it is an important aspect of what may be happening in a Zero Balancing session. The eight extraordinary vessels function as reservoirs of energetic power that are drawn on in times of stressful overload. They are a bridge between our pre-natal formation and the unfolding of our post-natal development. Their pathways form a matrix field that can be visualised in the form of a vertical egg, enveloping and nurturing us. Whereas the 12 meridian pathways are given a relationship with our visceral organs, the eight extraordinary vessels have a particular connection with our bones, bone marrow and brains. They are recognised as being instrumental in the fundamental cycles of life and hormonal changes.

Whilst we begin to stand upright on two feet with our spine vertical usually by the end of our first year of life, it is not until later in our teens that we stand on our two feet and fully take our stance in the world, having grown up. The freely moveable joints of our opposable thumbs are under our voluntary control. The talo-calcaneal joint, being a foundation joint, works at a different level of awareness. The use of our thumb with our hand in combination with our brain and eyes is frequently cited as key to our human development. The ankle in relation to the understanding of the Qiao Mai uniting of foot, brain and eye needs similar recognition in our human development. Both allow rich possibilities of movement as they are known as 'universal joints'. The development of our hands gives us comprehension. The development of standing upright on our own two feet give us understanding.

Another Chinese reference to the significance of power of this area of the body is contained in the writings of the Chinese Daoist philosopher Zhuang Zi. He writes that 'the authentic man breathe through his heels', which is comprehensible once these energetics of the body are appreciated.

Zero Balancing has the potential to reconnect us with the primal unity of our core structure and energy in profound ways that are beyond words, empty and marvellous. Some of the wonder of this is that it does so with apparently minimal effort on the part of the Zero Balancer. This is a sign that something is happening which is marvellous, well regulated and extraordinary.

The eight extraordinary vessels restore, regenerate and return. I recognise the sense of returning to primary origin as an important potential benefit in Zero Balancing.

This half moon vector opens and closes the journey that can be a Zero Balancing session. The two legs are being held equally. Through the two, the structural energetic central unity of the body as one can manifest. The two returns to the one and to the zero within. This is a subject I explore in Chapter 14 later.

9

The Dorsal Hinge

I n the middle of our trunk lies an important area between the thoracic and abdominal cavities and the thoracic and lumbar vertebrae known as the dorsal hinge. It is a good example to take in exploring the structural energetic anatomy in Zero Balancing.

The dorsal hinge is a vital bridge of transition in the centre of our trunk. The way in which it is in a dynamic balance can have implications for how we are functioning elsewhere in our whole trunk and body-mind.

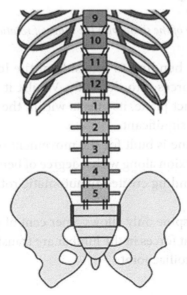

Schematic posterior view of the back with intervertebral facet relationships

The construction of the thoracic vertebrae means that they have an oblique facet between each of the vertebra. This allows a good degree of pure rotatory movement, up to 35 per cent. Further rotational movement is restricted by the sternum. Flexion is limited by the ribs and sternum. Bending backwards in extension is limited by the spinous processes of the vertebrae. Lateral flexion or side bending is limited by the rib cage and sternum.

The relationship of the lumbar vertebrae to each other reveals a different structure. Their facets are vertical. This means that pure rotational motion in the lumbar spine is limited to 5 per cent.

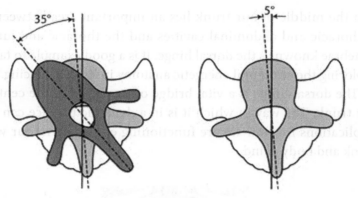

Overhead view of the spine with the range of rotational movement

Lateral flexion or bending to one side of the lower trunk brings a complexity of forces into the body. Whilst it may appear to be moving in a distinct plane, its effects within the lumbar spine and into the pelvis are significant.

The lumbar spine is built for the movement of bending directly forward in pure flexion along with a degree of bending backwards in extension. Side bending creates an automatic rotational movement in the lower back.

As the lumbar spine only allows 5 per cent of pure rotation, side bending means that forces in the lumbar are transferred directly into the pelvis and sacroiliac joint.

There is a key place of transition between the thoracic and lumbar vertebrae. This occurs at a vertebra where the superior facets are oblique and its inferior facets are vertical. This is known as the dorsal hinge. This is usually the 12th thoracic vertebra, but may vary in some people. Whilst this is structurally the anatomical centre of the dorsal hinge, the term applies to a wider area of functional and clinical influence.

Its immediate area has the lower ribs and 11th and 12th floating ribs. Muscular attachments bridge the hinge, providing support for the lumbar spine. The powerful dome-shaped muscle of the diaphragm defines the thoracic and abdominal cavities. In the front of the body lies the solar plexus.

The essential relationship of importance in Zero Balancing is between the dorsal hinge and the sacroiliac joint. Any movement of rotation or side bending in the upper trunk constantly transfers forces into the sacroiliac joint. The foundation nature of the sacroiliac joint means that tensions in it or misalignment can become held and difficult to free and clear.

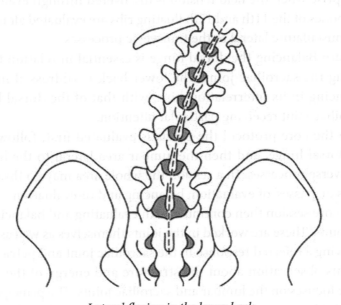

Lateral flexion in the lower back

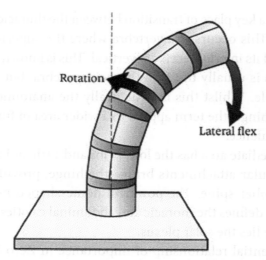

Diagram showing automatic rotation of spine in lateral flexion of lower back

A person may feel stiffness and discomfort in the lower lumbar and pelvis. Bodywork in this area can help alleviate this. The dorsal hinge area may be a place that is 'silent' to their awareness and it is a surprise when the held tension is discovered through evaluation. The bones of the 11th and 12th floating ribs are evaluated along with the musculature lateral to the transverse processes.

Zero Balancing the dorsal hinge is essential in relation to balancing the sacroiliac joint. The lower back is addressed in Zero Balancing in its interrelationships, with that of the dorsal hinge/sacroiliac joint receiving particular attention.

In the core protocol the pelvis is evaluated first, followed by the dorsal hinge, and then the lumbar area lateral to the lumbar transverse processes. In a session the whole area may go through a series of 'passes' of evaluation, balancing and re-evaluation.

A core session then continues with evaluating and balancing the hip joints. These are worked in the joints themselves as well as a way of having a referred response in the sacroiliac joint and pelvic bowl.

This observation about the structure and energy of the dorsal hinge focuses on the lumbar and sacroiliac joints. The principle that if a joint is compromised then the joints below as well as above may be affected means that it is also useful to consider the dorsal hinge's relationship with what is above it. This brings us into an awareness of thoracic vertebral articulation, the rib articulations and the diaphragm and the structural energetic functioning of the thoracic cage. A further exploration of this is available in the practical Zero Balancing part of this book (see the 'Metal element' section in Chapter 12).

10

Zero Balancing the Pelvic and Shoulder Girdles

We live in the core of our body – our trunk, spine and head.
Our limbs provide the means by which we interact with the world.
The two girdles connect these two through their structure and function.
The pelvic girdle is built for stability and the shoulder girdle for flexibility.

This chapter outlines a description of practical work which explores Zero Balancing the structure and energy of this anatomy. This selection of fulcrums, specifically designed to address the two girdles, are then fully integrated with the whole body in a complete Zero Balancing session. The sequence follows the order of a study day presentation for Zero Balancers.

Opening Evaluation of the Shoulder Girdle

The shoulder girdle consists of the two bones of the scapula and clavicle. It rests lightly on the top of the trunk, having only one bone articulation of the clavicle with the sternum. It is built for freedom of movement, retaining its stability through muscular and tendon connections.

With the client sitting on the side of the ZB table, the Zero Balancer stands behind them. In a Core Zero Balancing session the client's arm is taken through posterior circumduction with a focus on observing variations in their glenohumeral joint, as this can reveal potential restrictions in the semi-foundation joint articulations of the ribs with the thoracic vertebrae. This evaluation can also be used to give information about the shoulder girdle.

In this evaluation the Zero Balancer places their hand so that it rests on the client's shoulder, slightly covering the scapula with the middle finger towards the clavicle. The hand of the Zero Balancer holds the client's forearm, cradling it just distal to their elbow. The client is encouraged to let their arm rest in the supportive hold of the Zero Balancer and let them move their arm several movements circumduction. The scapula floats upon the upper back and the acromioclavicular joint articulates it with the clavicle. Both sides of the body are evaluated and it is possible to read the whole girdle movement as well as any asymmetric differences.

Does the shoulder girdle float on the trunk with stability or hyper-mobility? Does it hold tensions that the person has become used to as their norm or reflect particular use of one side of the upper body? Because the shoulder girdle is the transition between the trunk and arms, it can become affected by stresses which enter the body through the arms, as well as those coming from the thoracic cage, thoracic spine, heart and lungs, and the cervical vertebrae. Tensions from all these can result in restrictions to its freedom and ability to float on the trunk with ease and strength.

I give the example of a client who was unexpectedly dismissed from a responsible executive position in a charity. They had received no real explanation as to their departure other than administrative reorganisation, and had left without being able to train the person who succeeded them. They had played an important role in building the charity up and had 'put their heart' into the job with enthu-siastic generosity. One month after leaving, both their shoulders seized up, becoming 'frozen', which the person had never suffered with previously.

Evaluating the Pelvic Girdle

The pelvic girdle has the form of a bowl consisting of the ileum, pubic bones and sacrum. It is a marker of our maturing into full adulthood that it is not until our late teens or early twenties that the bones become one bowl.

The sacroiliac joint is the keystone foundation joint in the bowl which is the pelvic girdle. Its evaluation requires the Zero Balancer to place their thumbs on the client's sacrum close to the bony prominence of the ileum at the level of the sacroiliac joint. For the evaluation the Zero Balancer needs to be well placed in their own pelvis, as this stability will enable them to get a clear reading of the client's sacroiliac joints.

The Zero Balancer asks the client to rock from side to side, moving from where the Zero Balancer's thumbs are contacting their body. This not only gives information about the joints themselves, but can also reveal how the person is 'living' in their lower back, and their awareness of that area of their body. It can be that if the lumbar area and the pelvis become stiff and locked up, although the Zero Balancer has asked them to move from where their thumbs are placed, the client may actually move from their upper lumbar or dorsal hinge area rather than the sacroiliac area.

Pelvic Girdle Fulcrums

These fulcrums bring the three-dimensional circularity of the pelvic bowl alive through working with both hands of the Zero Balancer in an active relationship. The client lies down comfortably on the ZB table on their back.

1. The Zero Balancer contacts one side of the bowl with one hand nestling on the client's anterior superior iliac spine (ASIS) and the other in relation to their sacroiliac joint (SI). Taking out loose play and taking up slack, compress the ASIS downwards whilst bringing the SI fulcrum into mutual play. Feel the working relationship and connection between the two and the circularity of the pelvic bowl. Hold and then release. Go to the other side of their pelvis and repeat.

2. Inform the client what you will be doing and, having gained their permission, ask them to locate their pubic symphysis, noting its location. Sitting beside the person's pelvis, slip one palm down under the client's lateral upper thigh to arrive between their legs and lower pelvis. Turning your hand, you will arrive where one or two of your fingers can be in touch with the base of their coccyx bone. Then place the fingers of your other hand so that you are on the superior edge of the client's pubic symphysis. With both hands in position, take out any loose play, take up slack and engage both bones. Your finger(s) on the coccyx might also introduce a slight half moon towards the direction of their feet. Hold both for a minute or so with an awareness of the structure and energy of their relationship within the bowl. The previous fulcrum was to the side; this is at significant places on the central line, back and front.

3. Then, locating both ASIS with the palms of your hands, the Zero Balancer nestles the centre of the palm of their hand, matching the bony prominence of the client's ASIS. If the ZB table is too high, stand on a small stool to help you to work at an effective height. Using the relaxed weight of your body to introduce fulcrums, press equally directly downwards on both sides. Feel the circular connection of the whole pelvis. This fulcrum has a confirmatory effect on the structure and energy of the whole pelvic bowl. It also engages both ilia in relation to their SI joints. Hold with constancy for a minute and then gently remove your hands.

4. Close with a half moon vector of the whole pelvis, cupping the bowl of the client's pelvis with your hands. The previous fulcrum has a lateral 'horizontal' engagement on the circularity of the pelvis that this half moon complements in its longitudinal 'verticality'. Complete with integrating half moons at the popliteal knee crease and feet to end.

Shoulder Girdle Fulcrums

The joints of the shoulder girdle are freely moveable under voluntary control. To remind the Zero Balancer of their own anatomy, they can locate their acromioclavicular joint by raising their shoulders with a slight shrugging movement, placing their fingers on top of the acromioclavicular joint.

It is also useful to move your shoulders in a circular motion with your fingers on the saddle-shaped sternoclavicular joint to feel the anatomy and movement of this articulation.

1. With the client lying comfortably on the ZB table, the Zero Balancer sits behind them at the top of the ZB table. To create a fulcrum, place one finger in the hollow directly medial to the acromioclavicular joint, in close contact with the bones of the joint. Then add another finger fulcrum at the top of the humerus spanning the glenohumeral joint. There is a depression at the top of the deltoid muscle which reveals itself if you slightly abduct the arm. This fulcrum is one which spans the shoulder joint, enhancing the connections between the humerus and girdle. The fingers are in touch with both the head of the humerus bone where it articulates with the shoulder girdle and with the acromioclavicular articulation.

2. Fulcrums can also be placed on the body of the bone of the clavicle and also at the sternoclavicular articulation.

3. A fulcrum on the body of the scapula is often welcomed and the bone in itself benefits from Zero Balancing touch. This can specifically benefit the subscapular space as well as providing a stable focus which in turn frees up the movement of the scapula on the back. As the scapula is capable of radical freedom of movement, to introduce fulcrums into the bone holds it in a momentary stationary placement. This complementarity may be liberating in a person's awareness and the comfort and freedom of movement in their shoulder girdle. I also refer you to the fulcrum in the centre of the scapula which is detailed in the 'Earth element' section in Chapter 12.

4. Introduce a fulcrum into the ribs close to the medial border of the scapula. The area of the thoracic cage that is usually concealed lies under the scapula. The bone articulates with the rib cage through being anchored by the serratus anterior muscle. This is where the meridian pathway of the outer bladder line lies, running parallel to the inner line. The significance of the points here can be seen in the important names that reveal levels of power and the spirit of the organ officials of the viscera in relation to different vertebrae.

   Take the client's arm by their wrist and place it over their upper chest, and hold it gently in this placement. This opens up the space under the medial scapula. With your other hand and fingers, evaluate this area of the rib bones that is normally covered by the scapula. Introduce and hold fulcrums as required. Return the client's arm to its normal placement on their chest. Repeat the same process with the other arm and under the medial border of the other scapula. Return to the arm, so both are touching, resting on the client's chest.

5. This fulcrum addresses the shoulders as one girdle. The Zero Balancer sits comfortably at the head of the ZB table behind the client using their body so that their power comes from their pelvis rather than just their upper body and hands. Place the palms of both hands over the lateral extremity of the girdle covering the acromion bones. With a comfortable nestle of your hands on the lateral sections of their shoulder girdle, take out loose play and take up slack, pressing the whole girdle in a downward direction. Be gentle in using your body by using the power coming from the lower centre rather than only that of your hands, arms and own shoulders. The movement is with a slightly medial movement so that it focuses at a point in the centre of the client's pelvic girdle. With this fulcrum it is also possible to engage the body of the client's first rib with your thumbs.

   Hold this fulcrum on the shoulder girdle for a minute or so. The client may drop into temporary shallow breathing or apnoea. Slowly remove your hands, taking them away from their body, and let them breathe naturally of their own free will. The client may take a full breath and then return to breathe in a normal rhythm. Then gently massage the shoulder girdle and overlying muscles.

6. Continue by touching the prominent places under their thoracic cage along the body of their ribs (known in Zero Balancing as the rib angles). Then hold and gently lift the client's whole rib cage, supporting them with your hands outspread and your forearms well anchored on the ZB table. Complete with a half moon vector to integrate the head and neck, followed by the sequence of closing half moon vectors to integrate the whole body.

   The mobility of the shoulders, arms and movements of the neck are complemented by the first rib. Whilst the ribs from the 2nd to the 10th are involved in the activity of breathing, the first rib is well anchored, providing stability at a key place within an area of radical movement. This under-appreciated bone and its foundation joint articulation is significant. Matthias Alexander, who developed the Alexander Technique, recognised its importance, particularly in the ease of our head posture. It is interesting to note how the shape of certain necklaces which have a flat breadth, worn around the neck on the upper trunk, externally echo the structural form and energy of the first rib in their adornment.

Diagonal Fulcrums to Integrate Both Girdles

The Zero Balancer stands beside the centre of the client's body, at a height whereby they can comfortably reach opposite sides of the client's shoulder and pelvic girdles:

1. Place one palm on the anterior shoulder girdle with the hand nestling over the acromioclavicular articulation.

2. Place the other palm on the opposite side of their body with the hand nestling on the ASIS of the anterior ileum.

3. Simultaneously take out loose play to the blue line, with gentle downward compression.

4. Having engaged both girdles on the opposite sides of the client's body, take out the slack in a downward direction and add a small degree of mutual stretching, bringing an awareness of a diagonal connection between the two girdles.

5. Disconnect and remove your hands from their body.

6. Move around to the client's other side and continue creating this fulcrum on the other side of their two girdles in a complementary way.

These fulcrums simultaneously engage both of the client's girdles, at the top and base of the trunk, introducing a diagonal configuration to their relationship.

Complete the whole session by introducing the complete sequence of integrating fulcrums in the longitudinal line of the body (see illustration on page 85), ending with a closing half moon vector.

11

Our Key Centres of Gravity

A fundamental aspect of our structural energetic balance is the three key centres of gravity in our bodies. We coordinate and balance ourselves around them.

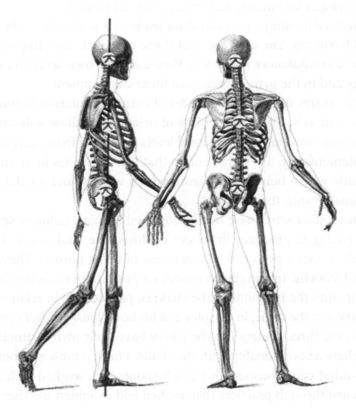

The three centres of gravity in alignment

These are especially important in the posture of our upright stance. They provide essential pivots whereby we maintain an awareness of living unity. We take them for granted but are frequently oblivious to their importance. They are hidden, forgotten and beneath our everyday consciousness. When did you last see a centre of gravity?

The three centres of gravity that are vitally important lie within the lower belly, middle chest and head–upper neck.

The basic protocol of Zero Balancing follows a sequence that addresses these three centres in respectful order. Each centre is balanced within itself and also in relationship with each other. This is key to the underlying harmony that is a fundamental hallmark of Zero Balancing. It puts a person back in touch with these centres, returning them to an embodied experience that has a sense of completeness. We are reconnected and reminded of levels of body-mind being. Our entirety feels thoroughly addressed.

Their awakening and unification leads to a well-ordered body-mind harmony. The awareness of these centres is also important for the Zero Balancer in the way they use their own structure and energy and in the path of their own inner development.

The centres of gravity are places of active orientation around a stable, still axis. These still points of orientation allow a dynamic equilibrium with multidimensional levels stemming from this paired complementarity. They are centres that can return us to an inner quietude whilst being places from which we conduct a balanced relationship with the world.

These vital centres have been recognised in many cultures' structural energetic practices that have explored the vital importance of their essential power to an awareness of being human. They are distinct from the Indian chakra model. Dr Fritz Smith made pertinent insights into the locations of the chakras, particularly in relation to the curves of the spine, in Chapter 2 of his book *Inner Bridges* (1986). Whilst the three centres I explore here have their own distinction, they share a commonality with the chakras in that both are about a body-mind consciousness that can be contacted, worked with and awakened through practices that awaken and enlighten us. They are also known in the internal work of the mystery traditions in many different cultures. Pioneering works such as *Hara* by Karlfried Graf

Dürckheim, published in the mid-twentieth century, revealed the cultural significance of the lower centre of gravity in both Eastern and Western cultures. There is clear recognition of their vital importance for a human being to cultivate their power in a coordinated unity. This is experienced as a living harmony of being actively alive whilst at centred peace within a form we are fully inhabiting.

The primary centre of gravity for our whole body is located in the lower abdomen. It lies within the body in front of the second sacral segment. This is a key area that is addressed in the basic protocol following the opening half moon vector in a Zero Balancing session. The sacroiliac joints are evaluated and balanced in relation to the lower trunk, pelvis, dorsal hinge and lumbar area. The relationships between the transitional lumbar-thoracic area are Zero Balanced in relation to areas lateral to the lumbar spine and the pelvic girdle.

After balancing the entire lower body, including the legs and feet, the Zero Balancer moves to the head of the ZB table and works with balancing the client's upper body. The rib cage, in which the middle centre resides, and the neck–head, in which the upper centre resides, are addressed in their integral interrelationship. This builds on the foundation work of having balanced the lower primary centre.

A Zero Balancing session is frequently completed with a sequence of integrating half moon vectors.

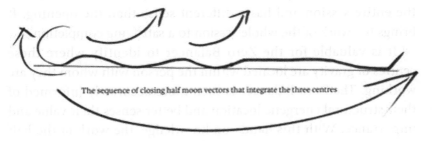

The sequence of closing half moon vectors that integrate the three centres

Half moon vectors integrating the head–neck, thoracic cage, pelvic girdle and whole body through the ankles

These half moon vectors align the body with the longitudinal central structural energetic flow whilst orienting the person around each individual centre of gravity. This unifies larger areas that have been balanced, integrating and coordinating their interrelationships, and bringing a whole session to a fulfilling completion.

The closing sequence of integrating half moon vectors begins with one to the head–neck. It confirms the orientation around the upper centre and the placement of the head naturally on the atlanto-occipital condyles with effortless support. When in balance our whole head floats on the spine in relation to our upright trunk without the tension you might expect, considering its weight. The flow of blood, nerve transmission and qi into our brain and senses is enhanced, and we are at ease in ourselves.

The next half moon vector in the closing sequence integrates the entire thoracic cage. The Zero Balancer places their hands so that their hold openly spans and embraces the whole of the back of the mid to lower rib cage. The half moon relaxes the person, re-confirming them in a central alignment. This lengthens and affirms the pleasure of living balance in this area of the body. It also connects with and unites the middle centre with the upper centre.

The half moon vector in the closing sequence requires the hands to be spread open and relaxed so that they can cup the bowl of the bones of the pelvic girdle. The lumbar spine and musculature may respond with further relaxation and lengthening. The client feels they have returned home to dwelling within this primary centre.

A session closes with a similar half moon vector to the opening half moon previously described. This closing half moon integrates the entire session and has a different sense than the opening. It brings the work of the whole session to a satisfying completion.

It is valuable for the Zero Balancer to identify where these centres of gravity are located within the person with whom they are working. The Zero Balancer is then more accurately informed of their structural energetic location and better senses their value and importance. With this hands-on knowledge, the work of the half moon vectors requires considerably less 'physical' effort, and so is not forced or a strain. They are then experienced as congruent with the relaxed power of the quality of touch of Zero Balancing.

The Zero Balancer is simply working with the client and orienting them around the axis of these centres, working with them in a way in which their structural energetics are naturally enhanced. It may not require much physical movement of their body. The half moon is placed in ways that literally remind the client of these hidden locations whilst they are lying in a relaxed horizontal position.

After they have arisen from the ZB table it can be valuable to ask them to simply walk up and down. This further aids the integration of the Zero Balancing session. They then inhabit their body, activating these centres in an upright stance, bringing all four limbs into coordinated movement.

For the client, this sequence of integrating half moons brings the session to a fulfilment. I am sometimes reminded of the cadences of chords in a classical symphony that signal the work's completion. The sense of being well composed and aligned in your centres can give an awareness of being naturally enthroned in yourself. Zero Balancing returns you to being well seated in your structure and energy. You are well centred and truly at home.

The Value to the Zero Balancer of Being Aware of these Three Centres

Lower centre

The practice of Zero Balancing requires the practitioner to work consciously with their own structure and energy. When they have an alive contact with their lower centre, the work of Zero Balancing is then practised with a relaxed power that has a gentle strength. They know and feel it and the client does too, with the myriad benefits of being worked with by someone at ease in their power.

When you drop your attention into your lower centre of gravity you activate it and work with your whole body. Your structure and energy is coming from a centred, balanced place. This is distinct from the strain that can occur if you only use your upper body and are disconnected with the roots of your primary centre.

Working with an alive lower centre is sometimes called 'getting behind yourself' in Zero Balancing, but is better described as 'being well placed within yourself'. Dropping into your lower centre activates the bones and relaxes the joints of the skeletal body. It gives a particular rooted power of being relaxed in yourself, manifesting in a gentle strength that doesn't require physical 'force'.

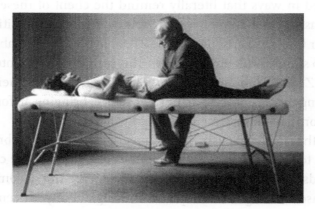

Fritz Smith Zero Balancing the sacroiliac joint

A Zero Balancer can find they are able to work for considerable lengths of time without tiring as they are using far less physical effort. This is congruent with a practice that is 'working with' the client rather than one that is only 'doing to' the client. The mind of the Zero Balancer is well rooted. Balancing originates from a centre within their whole body rather than their mind being confined to their head. Their hands are linked with their whole body rather than drawing only on the muscular power in their arms, shoulders and upper body.

The client's structure and energy responds to this by accessing a deeper level of relaxing in themselves. The quality of this touch engenders an instinctive trust in their working relationship with the Zero Balancer.

Middle centre

When the Zero Balancer is aware of this centre, their body retains an empowered posture and relaxed strength in the whole rib cage and upper trunk and arms. This gives them an alive connection with their body in combination with being rooted in the lower centre and providing a closer base to align the upper centre. Our vertical stance means that this centre relates us to the world in a totally different way than happens in quadrupeds. The externalisation of this centre can be seen in clothing displaying an identity or message, as happens, for example, on t-shirt designs or with jewellery.

This centre lies within the middle of the chest, at the level of the 4th intercostal space behind the sternum and in front of the intervertebral space between the 5th and 6th thoracic vertebrae. When this centre is actively alive, our movement does not compress our rib cage with subsequent limitation in our breathing. The arms and hands become natural extensions of the power connected to this centre.

This, in turn, is reflected in the quality and nature of the therapeutic relationship between the Zero Balancer and client. Holding the client in the highest possible regard has the meaning of recognising both the client's individuality as well as their human universality. This therapeutic skill is the foundation from which the ethical responsibilities of the practitioner are derived.

However, the virtues of when this centre is alive and awake can be seen in the level of non-judgement regarding the client.

The touch of Zero Balancing has an honest reality to it. It has a human directness that is distinct from any cosmetic, sentimental considerations. It has an objective clarity with a deep level of human respect. With this centre alive, the Zero Balancer's hands can more easily know how to be at the interface with the client. This distinction of touch in the working relationship of Zero Balancing gives the practitioner a body-felt awareness that they know where they end and the client begins, and the client knows where they are in this relationship. Any form of bodywork can generate an 'unearned intimacy', as if the practitioner and client have known each other closely for a long period of time. Zero Balancing maintains an objectivity with respectful relationship through the quality of its conscious touch.

When they sit up after a session, the client's structure and energy has been likened to clothing freshly removed from a wash.

The garments may need to be arranged so that any wrinkles or creases from washing do not stay and distort their true form. If there is a tendency for the person to sink their chest in flexion, this can affect the bowing of their head, moving it into forward flexion. Stand beside them, gently placing one finger on the front of their sternum at the level of the middle centre and the other at the level of their spine. Encourage them to breathe into their lungs and chest where you are touching, and their rib cage will then often come alive and fill. Notice the relationship of their middle centre to their neck and placement of their head. When the rib cage is aligned, move your finger gently to the top of the spine at the atlas, and the other gently on their brow between and just above their eyes. Allow the re-establishment of the middle centre to naturally align the upper centre of gravity.

Then ask them to carefully step down from the ZB table, contacting the ground with both feet, and ask them to walk a short distance. This actively integrates the middle and upper centres with the lower primary centre of gravity of their bodies.

Upper centre

The upper centre of gravity of the head is slightly in front of the atlanto-occipital joint. When this centre is alive, our heads rest effortlessly on the top of the spinal column whilst the head can move with flexible freedom. The central nervous system of the spine and brain is fully alive so that our perceptions and senses are consciously awake.

We pay attention to the activity of Zero Balancing, being alert and calm within ourselves. Awareness of the signs of working response in the client requires the development of the sensitivity of vision, hearing and smelling. Your hands are 'listening' through touch.

It is also possible in a session for the Zero Balancer to experience beneficial altered states of awareness that the client may also be experiencing. However, the Zero Balancer is acting as the responsible guide for the client in the rhythm and pace of a session. Pauses can have their importance without losing the flow of continuity in a session. It has a beginning, middle and end, and the Zero Balancer needs to be aware of where they are in this process. They are working within the relative world whilst simultaneously knowing that which is beyond time and space.

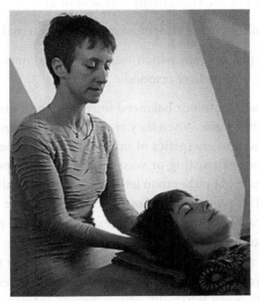

Zero Balancing the upper centre of gravity

Zero Balancing can develop an objective witness in the practitioner compared to practitioners who unconsciously project their personal subjective judgements. The clarity of the Zero Balancer's touch at the interface greatly aids the objectivity of perception, reducing transference and cultivating the ability to distinguish opinions from the accuracy of truth.

The Multiple Significance and Importance of the Three Centres

The awareness of structural energetic significance is implicit in many aspects of traditional cultures. Their importance needs to be appreciated on many levels. Here I select some of the most insightful, and give examples, particularly from the Far East:

- Centres of gravity around which we coordinate our movements and stance as upright beings

- Centres of the vital energy – as seas of qi

- Sites of cultivation and transformation in internal development

- Focal places from which our body-mind acts instinctively before our intellect responds

These are essential to our balanced movement and maintenance of dynamic equilibrium. When they are alive and coordinated we relax into the structural energetics of our being. We can be present and awake without exhausting or wasting energy, if we put effort into trying to be upright rather than letting the centres be alive in natural alignment. This postural effortlessness will be familiar to those who know the teachings of Matthias Alexander or who practise Taiji Quan or Qigong.

An alive axis gives us an active pivot that is key to the body-felt structural energetic experience of being centred. We are in the place allowing left/right, above/below, interior/exterior, to simply be in balanced relationship. A body-felt experience of axis as a pivot gives an alive awareness of dynamic equilibrium. It is a place where vertical alignment unifies with horizontal circularity. It combines the paradox of a still point around which movement manifests.

In the anatomy of Chinese acupuncture they are centres of qi and natural power. This has a quality of being in touch with a reservoir which, when activated, can be drawn on without depletion. When the lower centre is activated (often considered the centre of movement), we can feel a connection with a source of strength that may appear inexhaustible. For example, if you are dancing, it may feel like you could dance all night long without tiring. The Chinese named these centres appreciating their power as seas. A sea is a source that never dries up or is depleted. The etymology of the Chinese character for sea is *hai* (海), which includes the radical for water and of a woman who is lactating, with the meaning of mother, one who naturally nourishes her offspring.

When harmonised, subtle power is attracted to be within us. As centres of qi they are places where essences are stored and spirits can be attracted to dwell.

In many traditional Chinese internal practices these centres are known as places of transformational cultivation. The term in Chinese is Dan Tian (丹 田). The *tian* character is a field, a place where nourishment is cultivated. The *dan* character refers to a symbolic elixir. *Dan* in its natural state is mercuric sulphide, a red crystal salt known as cinnabar. When it is heated and the sulphur is burnt off, the precipitate is a dramatic transformation in both form and colour. The red salt becomes a silver-coloured metal of liquid mercury. This chemical change is also taken to represent an alchemical change of state. So, Dan Tian means the field of cultivation of the elixir, a place where profound transformation can occur given the right conditions.

In Chinese the character for transformation is *huà* (化). The etymology of this character is of a person jumping head over heels – a complete change. The Japanese animator of Studio Ghibli, the late Isao Takahata, showed such graphic transformation in his film 'Pom Poko'.

These sites in our body-mind can be recognised as functioning on an instinctive level. An instinct is an alive question that is always being asked and answered, often beneath a level of intellectual thought.

Zero Balancing can become a bodywork practice of meditation in action, similar to the activity of the internal martial art of Taiji Quan or Qigong. These are clearly much more than mere 'physical exercises'. The practice of Zero Balancing involves cultivation and working with internal principles. These have a body-felt perception of structural energetic reality in which the three centres are implicit. To awaken them in a coordinated way brings the mind into the whole body, your conscious awareness in your hands.

The unity of the three centres

Zero Balancing can be recognised as a practice that harmoniously develops all three centres in active interrelationship. This is inbuilt within the core protocol of Zero Balancing. However, it is valuable to recognise that one centre may have greater dominance or may be out of active relationship with the others, which can lead to its own distortions and imbalances. This situation can occur, for example, in martial arts where the lower movement centre can be activated without an accompanying awakening of the middle or upper centres. A person may then have martial presence and mobile power but lack a similarly developed relationship with their fellow human beings. In other circumstances a person's middle centre may open their heart but be disconnected to any accompanying development in their lower centre. This may lead to a person being full of good-hearted sentiments but be ungrounded in the world, unrooted from the realities of a vital connection with their lower centre. In circumstances where the upper centre is taken as the seat of their intellect, it is then possible for this to dominate a person's perceptions whilst being separated in degrees from the other two centres. Theories and ideas may abound which are disconnected from the realities of being in the wider world and their fellow human beings.

The portrait of the Chinese Emperor overleaf shows imagery reflecting a balanced cultivation of three centres in harmony. The lower centre is represented by the belt. Please note the insignia in its central circle which has the elemental configuration which will be explored in the following chapters. On his chest is displayed the dragon image reflecting in this middle centre the relationship of the power of heaven with heart-mind and the nation he governs and serves. The upper centre is seen in the symbols on the front and top of his crown, revealing a ruler with a quiet and awake body-mind fully enthroned within a human being.

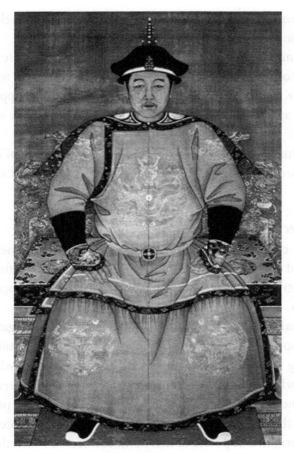

Chinese Emperor

The structural energetic anatomy surrounding the three centres, as found in significant acupuncture points

The knowledge the Chinese had of this anatomy is included here, with relevant acupuncture points selected to illustrate the radiance from these centres. This is to provide insight and information to inform our appreciation of their power and importance, rather than activating them through touch.

Refer to an acupuncture anatomy text if you need to identify their locations. The omission of charts in this book is because the limited number of illustrations and photographs were selected for other sections.

Acupuncture points are accessible in the soft tissue often in close relationship to the skeletal anatomy. The centres lie within our structure. Knowledge of these points can illuminate our appreciation of the still axis of the three centres manifest in our body's structural energetics.

It is valuable to appreciate the three-dimensionality of our body in the round, anterior and posterior, as well as the lateral sides.

LOWER CENTRE

The lower centre lies in front of the second sacral segment in the pelvic bowl of our lower abdomen. Whilst there is a specific location of the centre of gravity, its power and energetic influence cover a wider area.

Ren Mai 4 (Gate of Origin) – Guan Yuan – is the gate to our original source. The nourishment of our life originates here, combining the qi from the lineage of our inheritance with the qi from that which has nourished us since our birth. The *yuan* character (原) is sometimes written as a source of water, a spring of pure water issuing forth from under a hillside, or a source from a more primary heavenly origin. The power of this point connects us with that which is bringing us into a fulfilment of life.

A *guan* is a gate of importance that is a protected place of passage, like a border entry or a city gate. It is a gate with a central lock, allowing opening and closing as needed. The location of this point is on the anterior midline of the body in front of the lower centre of gravity. It is also usually where the aorta bifurcates into the two femoral arteries that supply both legs.

This point is mirrored on the spine between the 2nd and 3rd lumbar vertebrae of **Du Mai 4** (Gate of Life) – Ming Men. In the curled foetal form when we were in utero, the two points of Ren Mai 4 and Du Mai 4 lie at a similar level, back and front, as we were in flexion.

The Ming in Du Mai 4 is translated as destiny or the mandate that heaven has blessed you with – the inheritance that manifests as you fulfil your life.

Du Mai 4 is located in the space between the 2nd and 3rd lumbar vertebrae. A *men* is another door or gateway that needs to be able to flexibly open and close freely. Du Mai 4 is between the back *shu* points of the kidney and is described as the 'moving qi' between the kidneys. The 3rd lumbar vertebra is the central one of the five.

> The 3rd lumbar vertebra has a better developed vertebral arch that acts as a relay station for, on the one hand, the iliolumbar fibres of the latissimus as they insert into the transverse process of L3, and on the other, the ascending fibres of the spinalis, whose lowest point of origin is the spinous process of L3. Hence L3 is pulled posteriorly by muscles arising from the sacrum and ileum and can serve as the origin of the thoracic muscles. Therefore it is essential in the mechanics of the vertebral column at rest, the more so that it coincides with the apex of the lumbar curvature and its superior and inferior surfaces are parallel and horizontal. It is the first truly mobile lumbar vertebra. (Kapandji 1974, p.92)

Several acupuncture points on the central line of the lower abdomen have the alternative title of Dan Tian, the field of cultivation of the transformative elixir.

Ren Mai 3 (Central Pole) – Zhong Ji – is directly below Ren Mai 4 on the central line of the front of the body. It is recognised in descriptions of the eight extraordinary vessels as the origin of the inner central circuit, of the Ren Mai in the front of our body and the Du Mai that traverses the centre of the spine and head.

Li Shi-Zhen, the Chinese physician, wrote of this circuit:

> The Ren and Du Mai are like midnight and midday, they are the polar axis of the body… There is one source and two branches, one goes in the front and back of the body. When we try to divide these we see that yin and yang are inseparable. When we see them as one, we see that it is an indivisible whole. (Li Shi-Zhen, *Exposition on the Eight Extraordinary Vessels*)

Ren Mai 3 is in the middle of the body on both a vertical and horizontal axis. This is seen as the knotting of life in Chinese illustration, the interlacing of the combination of the two. Zhong Ji is also the Chinese name for the North Star in the heavens. This star is the one around which all others encircle. In time-lapse photographs of the night sky it is the still point centre, providing a place of stability around which all stars orient themselves. It is sometimes seen as the stand for Dan Tian, a place for pivotal cultivation.

Ren Mai 6 (Sea of Qi) – Qi Hai – reflects the power of the breaths when the lower centre is alive. The etymology of the character for *hai* (海), translated as the sea, combines the radical for water with that of a woman with lactating breasts, nourishment natural to a mother. This point is therefore the mother of qi, an inexhaustible reservoir that the whole body can draw on.

The greatest concentration of acupuncture points in the body (other than in certain areas on the head) is around the area of the lower centre in front of the second sacral segment. The fused vertebrae of the sacral bone has four foramina bilaterally, all of which are points. These are known as the eight winds, another reflection of the charged power in this area capable of movement in and orientation to all directions.

Stand beside another person who is standing and slightly curve one of your hands. With your fingers pointing downwards, place your hand so it provides a matching complement to cover their sacrum. Then ask the person to slowly begin walking forward. Gently and respectfully press your hand over the sacrum in the forward direction in which they are moving. This can often provide a surprising stimulus to their motion. Your hand is perfectly placed to contribute to the active movement of the lower centre in walking. When our movement originates from this centre, it has a power and coordination.

When you activate your structure and energy from this lower centre as a Zero Balancer, your work engages your whole body with a relaxed ease.

The rich multitude of points around the area can be seen in relation to the lower centre, but let me select one located laterally to the centre: **Gall Bladder 27** (Fifth Pivot) – Wu Shu. This is a 'wing' of the lower centre of gravity. It is a point on another one of the eight extraordinary vessels, the Dai Mai. This uniquely encircles the area horizontally rather than vertically, which all the other pathways do. Dai is a belt or girdle around the body, drawing together back and front, side and side. In the picture of the Chinese Emperor earlier in this chapter you will see this as an actual belt with the insignia of the original form of the five elements in the location of the lower centre.

The location of the point on the lateral muscles of the abdomen is worth noting. The pivoting around the lower centre activates the diagonal intermeshing of the abdominal muscles, the obliquus externus abdominis and the obliquus internus abdominis. They form a real girdle that is activated when movement pivots around the lower centre. This is important in the way this area of the body gathers itself in, the curves of the body in this area forming the waist. It is an example of the centre being the power that holds structure and energy in place. When the centre is a gathering point of the axis, this becomes potentially lost and forgotten.

MIDDLE CENTRE

Ren Mai 17 (Within the Breast) – Tan Zhong – is on the centre of the sternum, the middle of the chest and between the two breasts. The character *tan* in its left-hand part on its own has the meaning of being sincere, real and true. It is used in the name given to places of worship such as can be found in the name of the Temple of Heaven in Beijing, Dan Tian. The Emperor used this temple as a site for ritual observance with Heaven. The *tan* of Ren Mai 17 includes the flesh radical, signifying this as a bodily place of nurturing the awareness of conscious human relationships. In the centre of the chest it celebrates the circulation of the power of the heart and the breaths of qi with the lung.

It is one of the seas of qi that we also saw in the lower centre, Ren Mai 6. A sea is where the power of the breath has a focused gathering. There is also a relationship between Du Mai 4 on the lower back and Ren Mai 17 on the chest.

Ren Mai 17 has an alternative name of Yuan Er, translated as the Original Child, the character being of a young infant and the *yuan* of the heavenly source we also saw in the lower centre. This can be understood as the heart in the state of original open heart-mindedness.

All three centres are recognised as Dan Tian, places of inner cultivation and transformation.

Du Mai 10 (Spirit Tower) – Ling Tai – is located in the space between the 6th and 7th thoracic vertebrae, and **Du Mai 11** (Spirit Path) – Shen Dao – is between the 5th and 6th vertebrae. Both relate in the centre of the spine on the back at the same level as Ren Mai 17 in the front of the middle centre.

Both Chinese characters, *ling* and *shen*, relate to the spirits. *Ling* is literally the heavenly blessing of rain, the essential nourishment from above. The character has three squares that are three mouths of supplicants, dancing and praying for beneficent rain. The *tai* is a platform from which this activity might well issue. It can be translated as a terrace or stage, an auspicious high-placed look-out. The platform sutra takes its title from this as a place of communication with heaven.

In therapy work or Zero Balancing, our 'platform' is the ZB table. Here the client is in a safe place to be able to attract and receive the auspicious subtle power of the spirits.

At **Du Mai 11** the *shen* spirits orient the person on their true path in life. In Japan, Shen Dao is the name for Shinto, the indigenous practices of peoples of that island.

Du Mai 12 (Body Pillar) – Shen Zhu – is in the space between the 3rd and 4th thoracic vertebrae. The translation into 'body' may limit our comprehension to only our physical structure. It means not just our 'body' but also our sense of ourselves as a whole person.

When the middle centre becomes lost or weakened, the structure and energy of our posture can similarly collapse. This can be seen in the forward flexion of the upper body, not merely of the head and neck. It can be exacerbated by our sitting position such as using a computer when our attention is captivated and we become taken out of ourselves rather than being within our form.

The centre of our chest can become compressed and collapse, limiting the power of our breathing. We lose being well seated in ourselves, the lower centre disconnecting with a collapse of the middle centre.

When a person sits up on the side of the ZB table from having been lying down in their Zero Balancing, it can be useful to encourage their awareness of their alignment. Standing beside them, place one finger on their upper spine at the level of their back at Du Mai 12 and a finger of your other hand at the centre of their sternum around Ren Mai 17. Encourage them to breathe into the place in the centre of their chest where you are gently touching them. This sea of qi fills with a consequential lengthening of their spine and, in turn, the comfortable alignment of their head–neck.

There are also important points lying either side of the central pathways on both the front and back of our bodies, which manifest the power of the middle centre.

On the front of the chest, immediately above and either side of Ren Mai 17, lie **Kidney 24** (Spirit Burial Ground) – Ling Xu – and **Kidney 25** (Spirit Storehouse) – Shen Cang. These both have the characters *ling* and *shen* for spirit that we have seen previously. Ling Xu speaks of when the ability to be in contact with the refreshment from heaven has become buried. Shen Cang refers to our ability to have a place where the spirits can be rooted and stored within us. When the middle centre is active we can have a sense of the power of heaven enthroned in ourselves.

In the earlier picture of the Chinese Emperor on his throne, the image on the middle of his chest is of the symbol of the image of the dragon.

Either side of the middle of the spine, in relation to the middle centre, lie points on the bladder pathway, on both inner and further lateral lines. At the level of the intervertebral spaces between the 5th and 6th thoracic vertebrae is a point in direct correspondence with the heart and at the same level on the outer line: **Bladder 44** (Spirit Hall) – Shen Tang. This is a place of reception and housing for the spirits.

Moving to the anterior side of the body in a place locatable on a male body and covered by a woman's breast, we find **Heart Master 1** (Celestial Pool or Heavenly Pond) – Tian Chi. This is also the name used for the pool in which the magnetically charged needle of a Feng Shui compass floats. This reflects the power of heaven manifesting in the heart. It is essential to allow free orientation in relation to the world so the heart can circulate the natural joy and good spirit to the entire body.

On the lateral sides of the rib cage lies **Spleen 21** (Great Embracement) – Da Bao, the great embracement of the rib cage as it protects the heart and lungs, enveloping the middle Dan Tian. The rib cage needs to be able to respond to the movements of inhalation and exhalation. In the Jing Luo of the warp and weft of our structural energetic fabric, Spleen 21 is a point known for uniting the horizontal interconnections of the matrix of the *luo*. If you speak the point name in Chinese you hear its nature. Da (pronounced Dah) sounds the expansive power of great, the character showing a person standing with arms horizontally stretching out to both sides of their body. Bao (pronounced bough) complements the width of Da with a sound that captures the meaning of a container that envelops and protects whilst having alive interconnection:

> *The vital essence of things:*
> *It is this that brings them to life.*
> *It generates the five grains below*
> *And becomes the constellated stars above.*
> *When flowing amid heaven and earth,*
> *We call them the spirits or earth and heaven.*
> *When stored within the chest of a human being*
> *We call them sages.*
>
> *(Opening lines of* Nei Yeh, *an important early Chinese meditation text from the classic* Guan Zi)

UPPER CENTRE

The upper centre of gravity is located just in front of the atlas, C1, at the top of the spine. When the head is placed in relation to this axis, it sits with comfort and ease. The movement of free rotation from side to side as well as flexible flexion and extension becomes a secure place of orientation.

The considerable weight of the head is supported with a sense of it floating at ease on the top of the spinal column. We are vertical beings, and our upright stance means our head and senses have a distinct structural energetic relationship to the world, different to a quadruped. Our head is close to the sky and heavenly influence.

Du Mai 16 (Wind Palace) – Feng Fu – is located on the central line of the spine, between the atlas and the occiput. This is where the spine enters into the head, connecting with the brain.

In health, wind is synonymous with the primary power of the subtle qi by which we know the breaths of heaven. In the pathological context in Chinese medicine, wind is an external destabilising force, leading to disturbance such as constrictive stiffness and restrictive blockage.

Du Mai 16 is a point of dynamic animation to the head on many levels. If there is any misalignment or constriction, there can be a disturbance to our brains and senses or a held tension at the very top of our necks. When tensions rise upward in our bodies and are not cleared or freed, they can congeal in the structure and energy of our upper trunk and at the top of our necks, blocking the free transmission of nerves and qi flow into our brains.

Chapter 2 of the *Nei Jing Ling Shu* lists a series of points known collectively as 'windows of heaven', of which Du Mai 16 is one. Many of these points are located on the neck and all are involved with the relationship of qi connecting the trunk with the head-brain senses on multiple levels of functioning, including conscious awareness.

One of the alternative names for Du Mai 16 is Xing Xing. This character combines those for the heart with the stars in the heavens. It is the same character repeated twice, which gives a similar sound to that of the chirping of birds, a call that alerts you. Xing Xing can have a meaning of 'clearheadedness', of being astute, aware and consciously awake.

As the painter Francis Picabia said, 'Our heads are round in order for our thoughts to change direction.'

Either side of Du Mai 16 at the base of the occiput lies **Bladder 10** (Heavenly Pillar) – Tian Zhu – which holds up the globe of the head, like Atlas in Greece, giving it a place for it to rest securely and at ease.

In Zero Balancing, the head is evaluated in the full range of movements of the whole neck and also in the movement in the upper cervical spine. After an evaluation the head is routinely given a half moon vector that seats it in its relation to the spine. Lowering the head carefully so that the saucer-shaped occipital condyles rest on those of the atlas with a very slight hint of half moon flexion confirms the upper centre whilst aligning the head–neck with the spine and central flow. When meditators in a sitting position very slightly tuck their chin in to align their head, they are activating this connection.

If you gently press in the musculature at the base of the occiput either side of the spine, whilst keeping the head still, move your eyes and you can sometimes feel their movement under your fingers. Also, when you move your head on its centred seat in a gentle movement of slight flexion and extension, you can feel the relationship between the back and front of the head.

There are points that are relevant to appreciating these connections. One would be **Bladder 1** (Bright Eyes) – Jing Ming, the bright illumination of the eyes. This point was also referred to earlier (see Chapter 7). Between and very slightly above the eyes on the central flow of the Du Mai as it comes down the front of the head is **Yin Tang**, an 'extra' point on the Du Mai pathway.

This is the place of interconnection of the back and front of the body that also relates the cerebellum with the frontal lobes of the brain. Yin Tang is called the Hall (*tang*) of impressions. The *yin* character has the meaning of the placement of an official seal, a mark of identification.

Daoist exercises, such as the practice of *The Turtle*, mimic the natural movements made by the turtle's head and neck, to enliven the upper centre of gravity. I also encourage readers to look at the section in Dr Fritz Smith's *Inner Bridges* (1986, pp.161–4) on the venturi tube in relation to nasal passages and keeping your sinuses clear. The interconnection between the upper centre of gravity and the frontal lobe area is of considerable significance. There are many practices found in the movement and inner traditions of world cultures which illuminate the three centres individually and also reconnect them in balanced inter-relationship. The Japanese practice of Misogi breathing, whereby the upper centre is connected with and rooted in the lower centre, is an example that can awaken a living awareness of profound body-felt unity. The Japanese call the lower belly, which houses the lower centre of gravity, the *hara*. If the name hara is spoken, pronouncing it with a long a, you naturally connect with your lower centre through your intonation.

12

Qi Energy as the Breaths of Life

The Chinese character that graces the cover of this book has the Romanised translation of qi (氣). The sound made of its pronunciation is of an exhaled breath.

Its etymology can be explained as follows. The first stroke is of the movement of the atmosphere, as in the wind. At the top of the character are horizontal strokes with a curved stroke to their left. This shows steam rising upwards, like curling vapour. At the bottom centre left is the character for rice composed of a vertical and horizontal cross at its centre with four strokes. This can be interpreted as showing an inner crossing with the four diagonal strokes denoting the four quarters of north, south, east and west. The cooking rice bursts the container of the grain's hull and becomes food for everyone. The steam is the expanding aroma of rice cooking. Qi is describing essential nourishment as well as being used to mean the wider circulation of vapour arising to form clouds, with meanings related to the atmosphere and weather. It is both something that rebuilds us and the energy that gives us in our continual reformation. Touch can also be essential for our nourishment.

In a broad sense, everything can be seen as qi in varying qualities and number. The fundamental distinction within qi is the two complementary aspects. The fundamental expression of this is seen in yin and yang, the sunny and shaded sides of a mountain. It needs to be remembered that it is a single mountain and yin and yang are the double aspects of the one.

In the West it is easy for the term 'energy' to be taken for the active excitement of the yang aspect of qi. We can fail to realise the primary manifestation of qi as a complementary pair. The Western mind does not breathe!

> To facilitate the understanding of acupuncture by Western minds, early on in Europe we abandoned the notion of the breaths in favour of energy, presumed to be clearer. This doubtless obscured the meaning of many texts, created false problems, and accumulated forced and pointless explanations. It also narrowed the field of acupuncture and finally replaced a vision of man by a study of the physics of corporeal life. (Larre, Schatz and Rochet de la Vallée 1986, *Survey of Traditional Chinese Medicine*, p.51)

In the bodywork approach of Zero Balancing, the complementarities, for working purposes, are structure and energy in our bodies. Structure can be regarded as everything that is in relative stability and energy as everything that is in relative movement. Zero Balancing is characterised by having a focus on touching the most stable, firm structure in our body, our bones. Energy can range from the palpable rhythms within us to the subtlest forces of that which is bringing our life into being. Bone is an alive tissue, continually renewing itself with the potential to adapt to changes in our activities and the way forces influence our body.

Our energy body can extend beyond the parameters of our physical form. We can feel the warmth of the body's heat inches from the surface of the skin. This energy is visually evident in thermographic images of our body. Our structural and energetic bodies are not total matches; indeed, in states of imbalance they can become uncoupled, disturbed to incoherence.

13

Understanding Energy through the Five Elements

A formative time in the development by Dr Fritz Smith of Zero Balancing occurred when he was studying traditional acupuncture with J.R. Worsley in the early 1970s. Both acupuncture and Zero Balancing are practices that touch our structural energetics, whereby energy becomes alive and tangible.

Fritz's interest in studying acupuncture had been sparked by seeing J.R. Worsley at a seminar at the Esalen Institute in California. When he saw a patient being examined and treated and the insights into their condition, he was intrigued: 'Where is he getting his information from?' The description of J.R. Worsley's treatment and Fritz's response is recorded in Fritz's book *Inner Bridges* (1986).

J.R. Worsley was a pioneering practitioner and teacher who opened the door to the knowledge and practice of fundamental aspects of acupuncture. His teaching inspired several generations of practitioners in the UK and USA. He drew on classical traditions, and his approach became known as five-element acupuncture. Through skilful clinical application he demonstrated an approach that brought ancient wisdom alive in our own culture and time, and profoundly served patient needs.

One of the jewels of his teaching was to bring qi energy alive in nature and human beings through the insights of the five elements. This both theoretically and practically demonstrated how the unity of our body-mind-spirit health had to be understood in the wider ecological balance of the natural world.

The teachings of J.R. Worsley had a practical body-felt awareness of qi energy in our structure and energy. He opened the door to comprehend qi so you could 'get a handle on' energy and develop your skills across the wider range of your senses. For Fritz this was particularly important in awakening a new quality of touch sensitivity in coordination with other accompanying sensibilities. This was an important step on a path, one of unfolding development.

The cultivation of senses with elemental insight meant the practitioner looked beyond the surface appearances to perceive an inner dynamic. The underlying roots of imbalance became evident, helping the practitioner see beyond the presenting complaints. The universal was revealed in the individual. Treatment addressed the patient in a truly holistic way to return them to full health.

> The good point about the Worsley school is that JR has been able to put the emphasis on the knowledge of the Self of each patient and around that he has built a lot of things he has drawn from the Chinese tradition. Everybody knows that his strong point is that he is able to isolate, by means of his perception, the nature of the patient, and being full of strength is able to do a very impressive treatment. (Claude Larre, 1989, in a seminar on 'The Kidneys')

The Sense of Touch

J.R. Worsley frequently touched those he was examining in several ways. The pulses on both wrists were always palpated before, during and at the end of a treatment as feedback to assess the response. Several areas of the patient's body were routinely touched, such as the front of the main body as well as locally and distally, in areas requiring attention. His hands gained information directly, developing rapport with the patient and letting them know they were being 'seen' through being properly handled. The skills required to locate acupuncture points needed knowledge of the anatomy, along with a touch sensitivity to these places of access which are spaces. This was touching structure and energy with sensitivity and respect.

Chinese pulse reading palpates arteries, most frequently the radial artery at the wrist. The practitioner is feeling both the blood moving through the artery (the structure) and 'what is moving the blood', its rhythm and quality (its energy).

The touch developed in Zero Balancing brings you into contact with the person's structure and energy with a focus on their bones and joints, simultaneously reading the qi energy of their body, the most solid, stable body tissue of bone and the fluctuating vibratory rhythms of 'energy'. This is a fundamental paired couple.

These pairings in Chinese medicine include those of hot/cold, interior/exterior and the fundamental couple of yin/yang. The familiar symbol for yin/yang graphically displays the meaning of their characters, which is of the light and dark of the sunny and shady sides of a mountain. These are ever-changing areas, depending on the time of day. Whilst two fundamental qualities can be distinguished, it is essential to remember that the mountain is *one*.

Perceiving the unity of 'energy' at this level of two as a couple with complementary aspects is an insight intrinsic to the classical Chinese understanding of the world. The unity of the world was seen manifesting with greater richness such as human beings in their relationship between heaven and earth – the three.

The Significance of Numbers

One of the underlying ways of appreciating qi energy in the Chinese traditions is the hidden way energy is classically structured by seeing its integral unity at different levels of complexity. The nature of this unity is expressed through numbers and the relationships between them at differing levels. The one can be perceived at any level of complexity, all the way up to 10,000 beings, the number of the innumerate. Numbers have both a numerical quantity as well as the quality of relationship at any level of complexity.

A Numerological Vision in the Classical Chinese Traditions of Qi Manifesting

In the world of the breaths (qi energy) (氣)
That which is dispersed tends towards reunion,
That which is reunited tends towards expansion
The primordial chaos is represented by the one
One longs to divide into two whilst
retaining its unity as a couple
Two, the couple, longs to reunite around a pivot, three
Three aspires to spill out into heaven where it becomes
The four seasons and on earth the four
quadrants or compass directions
The dispersion implied by the four is attracted
to order itself around a centre, to create a regular cycle.
This is the origin of the five.

(*Claude Larre*)

At the level of five, the structure and energy of the world opens to reveal a wealth of information across time (seasons) and space (directions) and, within a human being, across multiple senses. This wealth of data is often seen compiled in five boxes of associated correspondences. Whilst this places them in their separate aspects, it dislocates us from the vision of their manifestation.

Information on the five elements is presented in the *Yellow Emperor's Inner Classic* (*Nei Jing*) in a systematic way in Chapters 4 and 5. Chapter 5 gives a template of how an element manifests in heaven, on earth and within a human being. This is the opening presentation in this classic of the Wood element:

In heaven it is the deep mystery,
In man it is the dao,
On earth it is transformation.
Transformation produces the five tastes,
The dao produces wisdom,
The deep mystery produces the spirits.
The spirits!

In heaven are wind,
On earth are wood
Of the parts of the body are the tendino-muscular movement.
(Yellow Emperor's Inner Classic, *Chapter 5*)

Chapter 5 continues with a detailed presentation of the correspondences associated with each element and their vital interrelationships. The first statement about each element begins with the quadrant of direction (space) from which the quality of qi energy of the element is characterised. The popularisation of the teaching of five elements in the West has often only emphasised the qualities of qi energy perceptible in different seasons (time). This has led to the importance of the direction becoming forgotten. The generative interaction of heaven (time) and earth (space) are then dislocated. The way the particular qualities of the elements manifest their qi energy within us as human beings is potentially lost.

The form of our bodies reveals an unfolding logic of structure and energy. In the bones of all our limbs, the upper sections begin with the one (humerus, femur), growing into the two (radius and ulna, tibia and fibula) and then into the five (metacarpals and metatarsals, five fingers and toes).

The Two Integral within the Five

Two, an even number, is perfectly complemented by the five, an odd number. They are both prime numbers, underlying the fundamental ways qi is structured and comprehended in traditional Chinese medicine and culture.

An emphasis on the five without the two and vice versa divorces awareness and practice in an imbalanced way. This has potentially distorted development in certain Western approaches to Oriental medicine. To know the two and the five transcends any schisms or myopic beliefs.

The (so-called) five element traditions need to be aware that the two is implicit in the qi at the level of five.

The characters for five and element have an integral rhythm of the two in the etymology through which we can properly understand their meaning. *Wu* (five) (五) was originally two diagonal lines crossing in an X. This showed the four interacting at a central crossing, then two horizontal lines at the top and bottom were added, graphically indicating above and below, heaven and earth. The character *xing* (行), commonly translated as element, contains paired components. These are left and right legs/feet, meaning a two-legged human being walking, our most fundamental movement. Walking is a progression of the coordinated motion of the interactions of the two.

Xing became used for wider meanings of movement that has an integral order to it. It has been translated as phase, process or element. You can see the way the West's comprehension struggles with something that can be perceived as structure and energy, choosing a noun or verb according to context or understanding.

Original Order of Presentation of the Five Elements

The first place in Chinese writing that mentions the five elements presents them thus:

> The five elements – the first is water, the second fire, the third wood, the fourth metal, the fifth earth.
>
> Water moistens and descends, fire burns and ascends, wood bends and straightens, metal yields and changes, earth receives seeds and gives crops. (*The Book of Documents*, *Shu Jing*, Hong Fan section)

It gives the awareness that what is being described is a vital inner movement of life that can be distinguished by distinct manifestations perceptible across differing phenomena. The order of the elements follows Water, Fire, Wood, Metal and Earth. Their elemental characteristics can be understood in complementary pairings – Water/Fire, then Wood/Metal, then all four gathered at the crossing at the centre in Earth.

Water is said to moisten and descend, Fire is said to burn and ascend. After these key opening statements, the element's taste that characterises its qi is given: Water and a salty taste, Fire and a bitter taste, etc. Taste as important to our essential nourishment is the inner movement of qi of the element. This awareness is vital in Chinese herbal prescriptions and the selection of food in its varied cuisine. Salt has a contracting action, and a salt crystal will attract moisture to it if you leave it open to the air. Salt is also the elemental taste that naturally assumes a form (prior to sugar being refined). The bitter taste of Fire found in coffee or unsweetened chocolate has a stimulating, warming energy, congruent with the activating nature of its elemental qi.

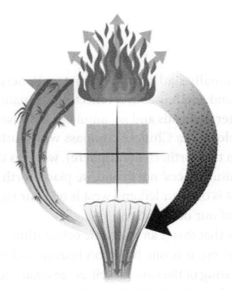

The energetic dynamics of the five elements

The taste of astringency is resonant with the elemental character of Wood's activating renewal. The spicy taste is associated with Metal, with the natural sweetness of Earth being the taste that covers all, as Earth does by being in the centre.

The four quadrants show the influence of qi coming from a particular direction, each element receiving it and giving it a particular characteristic. Water (north) and Fire (south) are complementary pairings, as are Wood (east) and Metal (west), with Earth as the centre, as it gathers all directions by being in the middle place.

The characters for the directions of Wood (east) and Metal (west), also show the expanding energy of the day's illumination and the withdrawal of light in the evening. The character for east is of the sun rising and shining through the trees. The character for west is of birds returning to their nests at sunset. The Earth as the central region is not a direction but a place or area.

In Chinese, Earth as an element is a distinct character to earth seen in the pairing heaven/earth, here meaning the world. Earth as an element is humus, the soil, the place out of which our nourishment grows. Earth in the couple of heaven/earth has a wider 'global' relationship.

Orientation

Chinese traditionally had its own structural/energetic logic, so north is below and south is above, reflecting the natural movement of their qi – water descends and accumulates, fire rises and expands – above and below. The Chinese compass was south-facing (even though it was in the northern hemisphere), whereas the compass in our Western culture 'faces' north and we place north above. In this orientation, east is on your left and west is on your right side, which is the opposite of our designation!

So you know that this is an energetic orientation with a radically different perception. It is one based on heaven and earth, the daily dawning and setting of the sun, as well as seasonal couples of spring and autumn, and summer and winter. It is auspicious to face south, the direction from which you receive the radiance that then radiates within you.

It should also be noted that, in traditional Chinese writing or printed word, you read from right to left and in columns, from top to bottom.

The Paired Couplings within the Five Elements

The elements each have a distinct nature with associations, whilst also being in relationships of complementary pairings: Water (north, winter, our backs) and Fire (south, summer, the front of our body); Wood (east, spring, our left-hand side) with Metal (west, autumn, our right-hand side). Earth, the crossing, is associated in time with the season of late summer, which can also be recognised as the transitional end of each season before the next season manifests. It is the central region as it qualifies all four directions.

This dynamic complementary pairing is fundamental to the awareness of the elements – seeing the two in vital relationship is a core awareness that is so integral to the classical Chinese mind it is taken as a given and can therefore be less immediately obvious to a Westerner's understanding.

The Qi of the Element Manifesting in Our Body

Each element gives rise to aspects of our body and functioning that resonate with the common quality of their qi. Whilst we may tend to focus on the structure, it is important to understand that it is both a structural and energetic manifestation, form and movement. When Water is associated with bones, this living hidden inner core of structure and energy is recognised as the way the qi of this element manifests in our body. In the original texts the taste associated with each element appears as one of the first correspondences. The taste is the quality of the qi inherent to its nature and movement and essential to the maintenance of life through cooking or in medicine through remedial prescriptions. The associations range widely over organs, colour, sounds, senses, emotions and odours.

This presentation of the five elements is a way of 'getting a handle' on the structure of energy for a fuller understanding of qi. They are not explicitly part of Zero Balancing practice but are of great value in comprehending the world of structure and energy.

This is an introduction to the nature of the qi of the five elements. Information has been selected from the classical Chinese insights to bring the energy and structure of the elements alive for Zero Balancers. This presentation complements existing writing for acupuncturists, and will also refresh comprehension of the elements in relation to this therapy. Zero Balancing has a focus on the pairing of structure and energy. The following presentation of the five elements emphasises the inner pairings within the five. An aspect of Zero Balancing work is explored to illustrate this exposition of the nature of the elements. References to Chinese characters are designed to illustrate the energy of specific elements, whilst recognising that these aspects can be observed in several different contexts.

Water element

Characteristic movement of qi: descending, flowing, infusing.

Body correspondence: bones as core structure.

Direction: north – our back, hidden behind us.

Season: winter – slowed down, cold, contraction.

Qi experience: fluidity – knowing the way to descend to the lowest place and to enter into the interior for core restoration.

Virtue of Water: ability to drop into deep interior to restore, the blessings of being able to allow water to support you – floating, letting go in alignment with gravity, creating a stimulation to the structure and energy of bone renewal.

Our bodies are mainly composed of water. It is essential for us to be conscious of and well connected with its nature. This is more than simply drinking sufficient fluids, but rather to fully appreciate this fundamental element of life in our body-mind.

In Zero Balancing this occurs early on in the sitting evaluations when the Zero Balancer picks up the client's forearm and moves it passively through posterior circumduction. The client is instructed to 'Just let your arm rest in my hand and I will make the movement for you'. Beyond the actual evaluations of the articulations, it can reveal how well the person is able to let go, give the practitioner their arm and trust them in moving their body on their behalf. It begins a relationship in which practitioner and client are both working together, mutually active. The client's 'activity' is to rest in the practitioner's hands, let go of trying, relax and enjoy themselves in an interaction they can completely trust in.

It is interesting that if people can relax their bodies, the 'weight' feels much heavier than their 'physical' weight should actually feel. If you are unfortunately hit accidentally by a totally relaxed arm, the power of its effect can feel greater than one moved with conscious tension. A person can be physically heavy but feel energetically 'light', and conversely, a person can be underweight but be holding the dead weight of tension and feel energetically 'heavy'.

The nature of working with this element can be likened to the skill of being able to float in and on water. If you are in water trying to float and putting in an effort to do so, further trying only increases tension. The more you try, the more you are likely to be unable to float and potentially drown. This is an embodied experience of the body-felt conundrum that is a double-bind 'activity'. The more you try, the less you float. If you simply let go and become one with this element, the better water will support you.

There is a tale in the writings of the Chinese philosopher Zhuang Zi of Confucius and his followers seeing a man apparently falling into a fast-moving river. Rushing in trepidation as to his fate further along the river, they see him emerge unscathed from the torrent. When he is asked how he managed this he says, 'I went in with the swirl and came out with the whirl.'

Being in seawater or a mineral-rich solution such as found in flotation tanks gives good support to experience floating. In particular, it allows the water to support the weight of our heads when we are lying on our backs, an act of real trust. This can also reflect the levels of unconscious tension we sometimes hold in our necks.

The qi of the Water element in our bodies manifests particularly in our bones. Our skeleton is hidden within the depths of our body. It has frequently been noted that the shapes of our bones reveal the flows and spirals of the forces that have brought them into their form. This reflection of the motion of water can be seen vividly in the form of the bones such as along the length of the humerus and fibula.

Bone is made up of bone cells, collagen and apatite. The inner structure of the formation of bone can be seen in the trabeculae revealed in X-rays or dissection. Bone is a responsive living tissue that is constantly being renewed and remodelled as it adapts to forces and to gravity. The collagen is responsive to electrical fields generated through compression or stretching, stimulating a 'piezoelectrical' current enlivening the structure.

The element Water reflects the power found coming from the north. The Chinese character for the north is *bei* (as in Beijing, the northern capital), and shows two people back to back (北). This is a position of non-communication such as you might find in the silent cold in winter, when life has withdrawn deep in the interior. Life conserves its vitality in order to survive and restore itself through the deep replenishment of returning us to our origins.

Our back is often an area of our body we rarely see and is therefore hidden to us. We are unconscious of our back and similarly the core interior of our bones. In Zero Balancing, our backs are touched and brought alive and into our awareness as fulcrums engage our backs whilst we are lying on them in a state of relaxation. A fulcrum becomes an invitation to sink into its support. The Zero Balancer's fingers have evaluated where they should be placed. With the client accepting the invitation, the fulcrum can then release tensions that melt and flow away.

Every bone is a floating structure, and the experience of Zero Balancing can be one of floating within yourself.

In the element Water, the kidney is one of its chief organ officials. The Chinese character for the kidney contains in it the image of a servant, the etymology of which is of a responsible minister in the posture of prostration. This position requires you to be kneeling and bowing forward, assuming a humble and lowly place or obeisance. This allows the sacrum bone to float and release within the sacroiliac articulations within the whole of the pelvic bowl.

The mysteries of water still fascinate contemporary science – where it all came from on our planet or water's internal structure and properties. It is an element that can exist in fluid, solid and gaseous states. A particularity of its nature is that when frozen solid, it is lighter than the surrounding sea it floats within.

Water has always been recognised as an element of central importance to the Chinese. The regulation of its flow in terms of rivers and irrigation during historical periods when water was out of control gave Emperor Yu enduring appreciation in history. The appreciation of the qualities of the nature of water occurs frequently in many texts. Water embodies virtues that provide a model for behaviour and reflection.

It can be poured into containers of various shapes and compliantly adapts to each without complaint. If you tilt a vase to an angle, it will maintain an inherent level of horizontal balance. It is naturally transparent whilst being able to accept anything put into it. It is capable of clearing and purifying itself, as happens when sediment in suspension is allowed to settle to its depths over time. It is soft but has the power to wear down mountains. It is very responsive to movement but can become a clear mirror when left to itself, revealing a true image on reflection.

> The stillness of the sage is not simply a matter of their saying: 'Stillness is good!' and hence they are still. Rather they are still because none of the myriad things are able to agitate their heart-minds. When water is still, it illuminates one's whiskers and eyebrows, and in its placidity it provides a standard so that the skilled artisans can take their measure from it. If the stillness of water provides illumination, how much more so one's spirit. The stillness of heart-mind of the sage makes it a mirror to the whole world and looking glass for all the myriad things. (*Zhuang Zi*, Chapter 13)

> It is because the mirror and water do not, in anticipation, equip themselves with cleverness that the shapes they come into contact with cannot but show themselves as they are: square, round, bent and straight. (*Huainanzi*, Chapter 1)

THE SACRUM

When fulcrums are placed on the sacrum close by the sacroiliac articulation, with the client lying on their back, it can allow the sacrum to 'float' in the pelvic bowl. As this is in the centre of the person, there is potential for this awareness to be experienced within their whole structure and energy, all the way up to the head and down to the feet. Here, in the middle of the length of the body and at this midpoint, it is possible for a person to rest and float in their entire body-mind.

The accurate placement of this fulcrum and the quality of touch are vital factors in whether this occurs, to be well placed in relation to the centre of gravity in the pelvis and on the sacrum close to the adjoining iliac bones. The fulcrum may benefit from subtle modulation of the proportions of structure and energy. Following its initial introduction with the Zero Balancer's hands well anchored on the ZB table, the practitioner holds the bone of the sacrum simultaneously with any pulsation of the energy flowing palpably at their fingers. Maintaining these both together, very slightly, they sink down into the ZB table, allowing a 'breathing space' for the client to drop into. The practitioner is providing support and an opportunity to experience the nature of Water in the power of this element within themselves.

> When the pelvis is not balanced, we do not have the upward thrust that creates zero balance, the sense of weightlessness that can be experienced in the body. When the pelvis is aberrated, it does not allow this equipoise, this tranquillity in experience that a balanced pelvis shows. The combined forces acting on a balanced pelvis are in a moment of inertia near zero. It is always dynamic in action, but the forces balance out to near zero. (Feitis 1978, p.54)

In the practice of Taiji Quan you may hear the instruction to 'sink and relax' as you are standing and moving, vertically upright. The Chinese character being referred to is *song* (鬆). This has a meaning of dropping down into yourself in alignment, celebrating the power with which water descends without resistance. This activity of non-activity allows knots to naturally untie themselves and release blocks and unnecessarily held tensions we may be completely unaware of. The etymology of *song* contains the radical for hair, here with the image of the hair unfurled, being able to move in natural freedom.

Standing vertically you are not slumping; rather, you are resting into the support of water. Water allows minimal compression. You are sinking in aligned relationship, connecting above and below, heaven and earth, through your living form. This stimulates a piezoelectric response, generating a bio-electrical flow that can benefit bone and bone marrow. You are neither collapsing nor being 'weighed down' by gravity; rather, the experience as you continue to move is of floating and a lightness in your body-mind.

You are literally 'well connected' and attracting the subtle to dwell within your being. The paradoxical nature of this is well stated in *Daodejing*, Chapter 26:

> The heavy is the root of lightness, centered equilibrium is the master of agitation.

We live on a water-rich planet. Looking at our globe from space, the vast area of it that is ocean is very evident. The source of the Earth's water continues to be a subject of scientific speculation. As is frequently noted, water is the dominant substance in the composition of our body. The salinity of ocean water and that in our own body makes for a good conductor of energy. Our fluid bodies easily translate wave forms that can restructure our body's particle orientation to be more aligned with natural flows. Water has a density and surface strength. It combines firmness with a lack of compressibility and a softness in its liquidity.

My fellow Zero Balancing student teacher and oceanographer Cyrus Rhodes observed:

> The Zero Balancer works with the semi-fluid solid. By applying traction and making a structural-energetic connection the Zero Balancer engages at the most fundamental level of the elastic inter-molecular bonds. By introducing a stretch into these bonds the water based molecules can absorb energy and vibrate at a higher rate. Putting in a complicated fulcrum can even induce molecular movement and rotation. When a focused fulcrum is held, the molecules are given time to absorb energy and vibrate to the point of breaking molecular bonds. At this point change

and working signs can be observed and the molecular structure reorganises within a micro-second. A release of energy and heat is felt externally. Lightness, clarity and new connections are felt internally.

Fire element

Characteristic movement of qi: ascending and expanding.

Body correspondence: blood and pathways of circulation.

Direction: south – facing the sun, the front of our bodies and relating to others.

Season: summer – warmth of sun in the fullness of its radiance.

Qi experience: warming and circulating to the whole body.

Virtue of Fire: joyful enthusiasm and elation of being in good relationship – rising expansive movement, establishing warm relations with others as well as living with a sense of our authentic selves. In combined balance with the downward rooting of water, the subtler energies are attracted to dwell within us.

Fire has a distinct movement of qi, which is the complementary opposite to that of Water. Fire rises upwards and radiates, expanding outwards. Fire and Water perfectly balance each other's nature. When Water roots a person within themselves, Fire can then circulate and realise an energetic harmony. This essential balance develops the conditions whereby the upward force of Fire is well rooted and will not blaze out of control. The potential volatility of Fire then has a place in which to reside. This integrity opens the possibility of attracting subtle energies to dwell with security within us.

The energy of the Fire element ascends and radiates. The glow of its rising expansive nature is graphically exhibited in the Chinese character *huo* (火).

The energy of life in our body can be felt from the rhythms and power of the circulation of blood animating life throughout our form.

We are warm-blooded and our thermal radiation can be felt beyond the bounds of our structural body. In Zero Balancing, attention is given to whether the person is comfortably warm enough during the session, and providing covering as needed to conserve their Fire.

In a session a person is lying comparatively still, yet Zero Balancing can stimulate good circulation even though they are not involved in the vigour of cardiovascular exercise. This manifestation of good circulation can also be observed as a response in the gentle activities of Taiji Quan and Qigong. You can be moving slowly or even just standing and yet, when your qi is activated, you feel a pleasant warmth throughout your body, even to your extremities, which may even have been cool when you began.

Following the gentle movement of vectors or held fulcrums in Zero Balancing, the perception of harmonious circulation through the structure can become quite apparent. The radial artery fills and pulsates as you invite energy to flow through the structure of the arm in the integrating arm fulcrum. The popliteal artery can become evident as you hold the back of the knee flexure and introduce the half moon vector that integrates the legs with the pelvis, lower back and rest of the body. The ankles may be held at the end of a Zero Balancing where your hands hold the person's opposite foot. The presence of the popliteal pulse on the inside of the ankles as well as the arterial pulse on top of the tarsal bones can often be felt pulsating, whereas it may not have been evident before.

We are in an active relationship of touch. This can feel surprisingly deep, and a person can feel significantly 'touched' in themselves.

Fire is reflected in the nature of relationship. As with all therapeutic relationships, in Zero Balancing this is conducted with respect and ethical awareness. Using interface touch develops clarity of relationship between you and the client, and they with you. It can give them an opportunity to recognise their own relationship with themselves. It is impossible to tickle yourself! However, Zero Balancing can reconnect you with your essential nature, allowing you to laugh at yourself.

The protocol of evaluation, fulcrums and re-evaluation involves working with touch, then removing your hands from the client's body followed by re-engaging again. This is quite different to some massage approaches where the practitioner is encouraged to maintain continual contact throughout the session. Zero Balancing allows the person to feel touched but to know who they are. Taking your hands off their body does not mean you are absenting yourself; rather, you are giving them the opportunity to respond for themselves. Combined with interface touch, this lessens potential 'dependency'. When you remove your hands, it is often prefaced by a gentle confirmatory squeeze, giving a non-verbal pacing indicator that you are removing your hands, which also affirms who they are and who you are.

Fire can have volatility, be lit, spark, and possibly blaze out of control. The possibility of injury to our Fire energy is there, especially if trust is abused, power taken advantage of or a relationship exploited. Fire is involved in the nature of a person's close personal relationships and how balanced their experience has been or how painful. Their body-mind may become guarded or unresponsive. Zero Balancing has a place in using touch to re-establish trusting relationship, and can be of service in situations of abuse. There may be degrees of self-hatred, defensive disassociation or levels of body dysmorphia.

The warm and respectful touch of Zero Balancing with the client also 'protected' in their clothing can significantly contact them, going beneath the layers of previous reaction or distrust.

We are warm-blooded creatures, and the warmth of Fire circulates throughout our body/mind. Whilst structurally our heart is a visceral muscle, the electrical power of the energy is considerable.

Fire governs the front of the body and the southerly direction from which the sun shines. With Water, the Chinese character for north showed two people back to back, reflecting being out of communication. When we meet and relate to other people we respectfully face each other. In a Zero Balancing session the client is lying face up and the practitioner faces them.

The outward expansive nature of Fire energy reveals itself in the nature and quality of our relationships. The interaction the Zero Balancer has with the client in Zero Balancing is of the greatest importance. Holding them in the highest possible regard and respecting their humanity becomes natural through the manner in which they are handled.

The nature of the quality of touch chosen to work with the client's structure and energy in Zero Balancing is that of interface. You are touching their structure and energy with your structure and energy. With interface the client knows where they end and you begin, and you know where they begin and you end. This develops skilled touch, which maintains a high level of clarity of relationship whilst working in profound ways.

In Zero Balancing it is possible that a person feels touched in a way that can feel profound. We are together with them for a short time, and yet feel we've known them for a long time. We have not spent years getting to know them, yet in a few minutes we are in deep and meaningful contact. The essential skill of interface touch allows us to work together with the utmost respect, and to meet and part with clarity and non-attachment.

As a bodywork approach, Zero Balancing is often greatly enjoyable, nourishing the sense of quiet, inner Fire.

An important response to Zero Balancing touch is that it activates the client's structure and energy, so that both of you are actively engaged in the work of the session. This activation is a rich working relationship. The working signs previously detailed allow you to monitor their feedback, which is often non-verbal. Whereas in many therapies you are involved in doing something to the client, in Zero Balancing you are working with them. This demands a particular quality of attention and a responsible awareness of being with them.

Confucius recognised a high level of relationship between people known in the Chinese character *ren* (仁). This has the radical for a human being combined with that for the number two. Representing human virtue, it is sometimes translated as benevolence or humaneness. The Chinese character for two is written in the same way that we write 'equals to'. The quality of touch and respectful way of being handled in a Zero Balancing session can be as if you are being met as a true equal, a fellow human being without comparison or judgement. This affirms both the virtue and importance of interface touch.

The quality of the qi of the Fire element can be seen in the nature of relationship. This might be in our relationship with ourselves as well as with others and the world. All hands-on therapy brings the beneficial warmth of human touch and can nourish our Fire. Zero Balancing has been found to particularly aid transcending feelings of loneliness or the sense of alienation – aloneness in the world. The fulcrums have a certain honest reality to them that through touch brings you into contact with your own nature. Our relationship with who we think we are, our individual and universal nature, is not merely a philosophical issue but also a living part of everyday body-mind-spirit consciousness. Historical identifications with who we are that may be better left behind can alter through skilful bodywork. When Zero Balancing is transformational, it can return us to a genuine sense of humour that allows us to laugh at ourselves and know who we really are. The fulcrums have a certain honest reality to them that through touch brings you into contact with your own nature. The character for the emotion associated with fire is *le* (樂), joyful happiness. The release and humour of seeing yourself in a new light is Fire being brought back to life within you. It has always amused me that it is not possible to tickle yourself. This is perhaps the double-bind of Fire that complements the one previously mentioned for Water.

Structure and energy in balance, Water and Fire, can give a body-felt experience of living unity. This harmony is an active balance of complementary opposites. When this condition is established there is not only a harmony of qi, but it is also an attractive environment conducive to awakening subtler energy.

Qi describes the energy in the relative world and specific functions. There can be multiple levels of the breaths. Health comes from returning to a unity of functioning regardless of their complexity. Perceiving the breaths of qi at the level of five is one that we can get a handle on in time and space. We have five fingers and two hands, which give these fundamental levels a familiar body-felt reality.

When the unity of qi is returned, it is then possible we may become aware of a subtler level that has its own nature and power. This may open us to beneficial altered states of consciousness.

The spirits are defined in Chinese culture as 'that which yin-yang cannot probe' (*I Jing* and *Nei Jing*). Our ability to perceive the movements of the relative world is no longer of use. Our normal perceptions of the relative world of time and space may no longer operate. Our awareness of what is time may feel different. We may feel distinctly different to our normal sense of our bodies, taller, freer. We may be lost for words – in a state in which language is not relevant or needed to be used. Inner quietude.

The heart as the organ official in Chinese medicine is translated as body-mind. The original glyph shows a bowl and openings for circulation. The bowl is an image of an empty and quiet mind, free of desire, complete and present, in control of the blood but in ways of ruling.

Love in this context is universal, not personal – we know that much-used word which has so many levels of meaning, yet only one word in our language. The indicators that it transcends the normal parameters of time and space are there in our common understanding of love. When we are in love with another we experience feelings of expansive generosity that transcends norms. We may pledge to want to be with this person forever, or share our possessions freely, all signs of altered states.

At the end of a session, when a person opens their eyes, stands up and takes a few steps, there is often a sparkle in their eyes. In Chinese medicine and culture this is known as the radiance of the spirits, Shen Ming (神 明). A structural appreciation of our vision is one of light coming into the eye. For the Chinese, the presence of the spirits within a person was revealed as light shining out through their eyes.

Wood element

Characteristic movement of qi: expansive activation.

Body correspondence: tendino-muscular forces.

Direction: east – image of the sun rising through the trees; left-hand side of the body.

Season: spring – the rapid return of life as the sap rises following the dormancy of winter.

Qi experience: smooth movement of well-lubricated joints – movement of bones and muscles in well-organised coordination; articulations – *jie* (節) – in both time and space – active vital movement as required by the situation.

Virtue of Wood: forceful power of renewal of life in spring and the start of a day. Release from frustration/restriction and events going to plan, whether this is smooth and unfolding progression or coordinated movement. Free and easy wandering in musculoskeletal motion as well as far-reaching creative imagination. The ability for decisions to be courageously enacted, adapting to changing circumstances in fulfilment of far-sighted, well-considered plans.

The structure and energy in the body is often best evaluated at the joints where the quality of movement can be assessed at the articulation. The structure of joints involves skin, muscles, tendons and ligaments. The latter are non-contractible tissue that provides an ultimate constraint within a joint, providing stability.

Joint movement can be measured by quantity of range of motion in relation to an expected norm. In Zero Balancing, reading the quality of motion is an important aspect of appreciating their structure and energy. Evaluation reads a joint in its normal range of motion, carefully taking it up to where the end range of motion begins to restrict further movement. Is the quality of movement too tight or too loose in the joint, in relation to its paired joint or in relation to other joints?

The forceful power of this element can be seen expressed in the body through the dynamic ability of Wood to move the joints freely and smoothly in coordination.

The Chinese character for the associated aspect of Wood in the body is *jin* (筋). This is best translated as tendino-muscular forces. These give connection between the bones and the flesh in order to make active movement.

Wood is related to the season of spring, the activation of the vitality of this element's qi bringing life into active motion. The character of *jin* contains the radical for bamboo, emblematic of firm, flexible, vibrant, growing vegetation. *Jin* are the fibres of wood within our form and function, stretching and bending with a similar nature. The character also contains the meaning of strength, and the flesh radical shows it is an aspect of our body.

In our youth the forces of our *jin* move us with vital suppleness. In our later years all too often this power of the qi of Wood can weaken, and our joints become stiff and less vital. Zero Balancing is valuable in maintaining our flexible strength and the precision of coordinated movement.

> *At birth a human being is soft and yielding*
> *At death hard and unyielding*
> *All beings, grass and trees when alive are soft and bending*
> *When dead are dry and brittle*
> *Therefore the hard and unyielding are the companions of death,*
> *The soft and yielding are the companions of life.*
>
> (Daodejing, *Chapter 76*)

Zero Balancing cultivates a relaxed strength in our body, maintaining the quality of the resilient power of Wood into our later years. The paradox of a body in this relaxed strength being 'stronger' than one being held in tension is an aspect of many qi exercises, seen in kinesiology testing or perfected in Koichi Tohei's demonstrations of Ki Aikido. Place your forefinger and thumb together and hold them in tension. Then try separating them in this state and when in relaxation. The 'strength' of good qi energy circulation through the combined joints of these digits when 'relaxed' can be impressive. When a baby holds your finger in its hand, it can be difficult to extract it from its grasp. This paradox is noted in *Daodejing*, Chapter 55: 'A nursing infant…though its bones are soft and its tendino-muscular forces pliant, and yet its grip is firm.'

When Wood is alive and balanced within us, it is not only seen in our bodily movement but also in flexibility in our mind and thoughts. We are able to bend with change, move and adapt to new circumstances with fresh ideas. I have seen the benefits of Zero Balancing in creative contexts, and it stimulates the flexible thinking required in problem solving – a composer coming out of a session and immediately going to the piano and writing music for a passage that had been frustrating him; a writer caught up in a creative block, then full of new ideas following a session. So many breakthroughs in the history of science have occurred following sleep. Zero Balancing can take a person into restful refreshment out of which insights and creative solutions can arise.

Zero Balancing evaluates the structure and energy particularly at the joints where the tightness or looseness of the tone of Wood can also be appreciated. It is possible to just select evaluation as a focus for surveying the whole person prior to any fulcrums being introduced.

PROTOCOL OF AN EVALUATORY ZERO BALANCING SESSION

It can be valuable to give a session that views the whole person's structure and energy with a complete evaluation before Zero Balancing fulcrums or vectors are used. These can then be selected so that they are customised to the client's specific needs. The evaluation gives an overview and discoveries that can have a satisfying integrity in itself.

The accuracy of well-applied structural energetic evaluation can provide a mirror for the person, taking them on a guided tour of themselves. It can reveal their overall condition and reveal where tensions are being held and the interrelationships between joints and areas of their body.

The Zero Balancer can survey the overall structural energetic tone of the client's body whilst gathering information about any observable asymmetry of paired joints:

1. Begin with the client giving you their own sense of their needs, their awareness of their body and how it is functioning.

2. Possibly initially evaluate any areas they highlight that you may explore further when they are lying down.

3. Sitting evaluations: first touch their back, discovering any palpable 'rib angles', moving from the top to lower ribs at a rhythm that brings them present. Then move their arms in posterior circumduction, closing with a waving farewell movement of the arm, known in Zero Balancing as 'Goodbye Charlie'. Note how well they give you their arm to relax into your hold and you work together. Evaluate their sacroiliac joints with the client in a sitting position.

4. When the client lies down, introduce the opening half moon vector. Use it as an evaluation of the joints in their legs and hips, how well they relax into themselves, how far up the body the vector 'registers', noting any 'working signs'.

5. Evaluate the sacroiliac joints and pelvis.

6. Evaluate the dorsal hinge and lumbar area.

7. Evaluate the hip joints.

8. Evaluate the tarsal joints and feet.

9. Introduce a half moon vector at the ankles to complete evaluating the lower body before moving to the upper body.

10. Evaluate the thoracic cage and rib angles.

11. Evaluate the trapezius, shoulder girdle and the movements of the whole and upper cervical vertebrae, noting their inter-relationships.

12. Complete this evaluation of the upper body by closing with an integrating half moon vector on the head–neck.

13. Then introduce a selection of fulcrums and vectors, and close by integrating this work with closing fulcrums. You could address the most essential areas first or, if following an order of Zero Balancing, work from the upper to lower body. Pay attention to the interactions between joint relationships as well as the client's responsiveness and sensitivity. As you move towards the end of this session, you can also verbally ask the client if there is anywhere they would like you to work on.

It is possible to complete this particular variation on a session within a relatively contained time of, for example, 15 minutes. An evaluatory session can also be useful in the context of a Zero Balancing workshop, where different areas of the body are being worked, and it is valuable to aid the assimilation of this work with a broader integration.

Metal element

Characteristic movement of qi: inward contraction.

Body correspondence: skin and surface tissue.

Direction: west – image of birds returning to roost at dusk; right-hand side of the body.

Season: autumn – the time of nature letting go of the growth of the summer and returning within itself.

Qi experience: fundamental coordinated rhythm of taking in and letting go the breath of life, inspiration/elimination – the bridge between voluntary and involuntary regulation of our structural and energetic functioning.

Virtue of Metal: rhythm in harmony, both letting go as well as taking in. Knowing what is of true value in life.

The quality of qi energy of the Metal element invites us to return within to recognise what is of real value within ourselves. Regardless of how much wealth a person has accumulated in their life, being in good health and alive spirits is of inestimable value.

The character for the direction from which Wood arises is east, the morning sun shining through the trees. The character for the direction of qi of Metal is the west, showing birds returning to their nests to roost in the eve of the day.

Wood and Metal are a couple, pairing expansion and contraction with their associated seasons of spring and autumn. These are the times of major transition between the polarities of winter and summer, and summer and winter. The early Chinese classic, the *Spring and Autumn Annals*, indicates from its title that its wisdom covered the entire subject.

The season of autumn that is resonantly associated with the nature of Metal for the Chinese is a time of transition from the full expansion of growth to a return to the interior. It is a time of reckoning, recalibration and rebalancing to what is essential to life. In financial accounting the term Zero Balancing means 'balancing the books'.

> In keeping the wood spirit and the metal spirit together, are you able to embrace their unity?
>
> In gathering your vital energy to attain suppleness, have you reached the state of a newborn babe?
>
> (Daodejing, *Chapter 10*)

The energy of metal returns us to inner regulation that in terms of qi is of a return to the natural vital rhythm of life for its balance, wellbeing and survival. Returning to being congruent with the circadian rhythms of night and day, spring and autumn is essential to maintaining our living balance.

Classical Chinese culture reminded society of the order of inner regulation through the whole range of the pure, clear tones of orchestras of metal instruments. The magnificent collections of bronze bells excavated from tombs in China reveal their importance in regulating and tuning, the musical equivalent of uniform weights and measures in maintaining standards and harmonic order in society.

Using metal to retune society is seen in the Chinese character *tiao* (調), translated as tuning. Tiao qi means to regulate or tune the qi energy in Chinese medicine as one might tune a musical instrument. Aligning and modulating structure and energy for optimum harmony is a good description for Zero Balancing. Zero Balancing can be understood as a way of retuning a person so they are resonant with the movement of life.

The title of Chapter 2 of *Su Wen* contains the character *tiao*, where it describes the importance of maintaining life by tuning your spirits with the qi of each season. *Tiao* is also found in medical classics as an appreciation of what essentially happens in the process of beneficial treatment.

The results of developing the practice of Zero Balancing give a practitioner the ability to instinctively 'know' the internal structure of where the bones and joints lie, concealed beneath the surface covering. It also touches their core interior respectfully, at a level where they feel significantly 'met' and 'touched'.

It bypasses the clothes and surface, entering into the depths of the client's body with care – to the level where their structure and energy can be contacted. I am reminded of other approaches, such as an acupuncturist palpating for where to enter the body, then inserting a needle and going to just the correct depth within the tissue, or a psychic surgeon, whom I have witnessed bypassing the surface to apparently go directly within the person's form with their hands.

Zero Balancing touch has an honest reality to it: evaluating with care, but not denying what needs to be recognised and addressed – what is there. It is not about 'being nice', but about being truthful. And then touching in a way that genuinely meets the person, going through the blue line, working with them. It is a touch that has a respectful firmness, that may become hedonic, but the person feels they are being touched where touch is really needed, in no uncertain terms but not into overload. It is working with them, checking in, and holding fulcrums as required.

Zero Balancing sets up the conditions where stronger energy can flow within and through our structure. We return to the experience of harmonic regulation. What may have been in the way of such reconnection is no longer blocking or adversely altering us. Its virtue has the nature of a clear breath of fresh qi in our body-mind and spirits.

The expression in Zero Balancing of 'clearer, stronger fields' expresses the refreshment of being reconnected with and retuned to the power of fundamental rhythms and vital relationships.

I am aware of an analogy to Zero Balancing in what happens in a technique to help make old recordings audibly clearer. The surface noise heard on vinyl or shellac can be removed by a method of first identifying what is extraneous to the original music or sound, such as the pops and clicks. Then a method is used by which a complementary match is found to these and is introduced, which neutralises and clears them. They disappear and the true music or sound can then be heard with clarity.

Zero Balancing fulcrums can clear what is in the way or is no longer needed, so that the person's real structure and energy returns and 'rings true'. This may take them into an inner silence where the previous cacophony obscuring their internal nature is no longer there.

A Zero Balancer may, whilst holding you in a fulcrum, say the phrase 'Let drop away that which no longer serves you'. This invitation to let go can welcome a release of tensions or beliefs that are extraneous to your present life.

The quality of touch in Zero Balancing is one of its essential characteristics. It is without judgement or extraneous agenda. The touch holds people in the 'highest possible regard'. Zero Balancing touch has a purity and clarity that allows the true nature of a person's structure and energy to manifest. Your essential being within you is being touched, through the layers of clothing or fascia.

In Chinese medicine the associated organ functions/officials of Metal are the lung and large intestine. Although located in different body cavities, they share a common aspect of Metal's functioning that is of essential rhythm, of breathing or digestive processing. They both take in and give out with an essential regularity of order that is their healthy functioning. Sometimes Zero Balancing sessions reminds the person's bowels of its normal rhythm of activity, returning it to keeping 'regular', as the phrase goes in the USA.

The description of the role and responsibility of the lung in Chapter 8 of *Su Wen* is pertinent in understanding the nature of the structure and energy of the Metal element.

When the lung fulfils its official responsibility, the result is the 'regulation of life giving rhythms' (Zhi Jie, 治 節). In Chinese, *zhi* (治) is to know how to live life. When *zhi* is used in relation to the body, it means to treat, cure or heal. It can also mean to govern a kingdom, because if you know how things operate, you know how to bring the country into ordered regulation.

The *jie* (節) is the character for the joints, described in the Wood element. It is a knot of bamboo, each knot marking an articulation in growth, where there is a concentration and from which there is another surging in a section of bamboo. Tuning one joint in relation to another fundamentally regulates the body's structural energetic functioning.

Attention is given in the practice of Zero Balancing to the pacing of a session, varying the pace accordingly and picking up the pace as required. This includes knowing when and how to 'pause', holding fulcrums with sensitive gauging of the 'space' the person is in. A session can be understood to have a musical nature. Silent rests between the notes are an essential part.

With our breath we take the air and atmosphere surrounding us into the intimacy of our lungs. We are in direct interrelationship between the external and internal worlds. Metal can bring us into sensitivity with the qi and the atmosphere surrounding us.

Freeing and returning breathing to its natural regulation brings the complementarities of inhalation/exhalation into a fundamental rhythm. This is the two as one, experienced as a body-mind unity. With this established it is possible to go from one to zero – not the absence of breath, apnoea, but beyond the two/one into a state beyond words. There can be times after the completion of a Zero Balancing session when the person sits up or steps down from the ZB table and they are silent when asked 'How are you?' or 'How do you feel?' They are not simply lost for words, but are in a wordless state. To speak takes you into commenting on, and you realise the limitations of language as an expression.

> *The Dao which can be spoken of is not the eternal dao,*
> *The name which can be named is not the eternal name.*
> *The nameless (non-being) is the origin of heaven and earth,*
> *The nameable (being) is the mother of the myriad things.*
>   (Daodejing, *opening lines of Chapter 1*)

Through an awareness of our breathing we can tune ourselves as well as with the living world. It is an activity involuntarily happening as well as one we can become aware of and voluntarily affect. The ways a client can respond to Zero Balancing are recognised through 'working signs', which include variations in the rhythms of involuntary breath patterns, previously referred to in Chapter 6.

As a person relaxes into themselves in a session, tensions in their diaphragm, intercostal muscles and rib cage can release. One observable response is that the whole of their trunk then becomes involved in their breathing, even though they are lying still and relaxed on the ZB table. There may be a movement in their abdominal muscles as their lower trunk plays its part in breathing, reflecting diaphragmatic relaxation.

Breath is an essential nourishment for us, along with food and water. The experience of being reconnected with the power of natural breathing can be liberating and refreshing. Our breath embodies the rhythm of inhalation and exhalation. We can also become aware of the momentary pause of transition between the in and out breath. This can be a window into what is beyond the two. When we are 'well ventilated', it is possible we may have the experience of the involuntary power of 'being breathed'. 'After a while I realised that the inhalation and exhalation of my body were as the expansion and contraction of the universe' (from the diagram illustrating inner meditation in the White Cloud Daoist monastery in Beijing). This speaks of the oneness of our being and the earth as a living planet which James Lovelock had in Gaia.

In Chapter 8 of *Su Wen* the description of the role of the lung is 'The regulation of all rhythms stems from it'. The character for rhythms is *jie* (節), the articulations or joints seen in Wood, but here given a wider meaning of regulation of life. These articulations can be in space, of our joints as well as in time, of the key 'articulations' of the year, the solstices or equinoxes.

THE DORSAL HINGE AND THE RIB CAGE

In Zero Balancing, the focus on the dorsal hinge at the thoracic–lumbar vertebral transition is in relation to the lower back and sacroiliac joint. It is also possible to see how the dorsal hinge can affect the structural energetics of what is above it.

The large dome-shaped muscle of the diaphragm is located close to the dorsal hinge above, and can be an aspect of held tensions in this area. The muscle defines the division and unification of the thoracic and lumbar cavities.

First, evaluate the area of the client's dorsal hinge in their mid-back. Then introduce fulcrums into the soft tissue and particularly along the body of the floating ribs. Hold fulcrums at the tip of the 12 ribs and then laterally, at the tip of the 11th rib.

Then locate on the anterior trunk at the inferior base of the rib cage where the 10th rib articulates. There is often a palpable notch along the line of the lower rib cage. It is often where the para-median nipple line would transect.

Then locate a place on the lateral side of the upper rib cage, just below the clavicle and medial to the coracoid process.

Place one fulcrum at the base of the rib cage and, with the other hand, a fulcrum at the top of the rib cage, and hold for a few seconds for it to register.

Then sit behind the person at the head of the ZB table and evaluate and work on the rib angles also in relation to the head–neck, to aid the integration of the previous fulcrum.

This might be followed by an interactive lung breath fulcrum.

INTERACTIVE LUNG BREATH FULCRUM

This is an interactive fulcrum in which the Zero Balancer gives the client clear instructions so that they work together. It is most usually introduced after all the work on the rib cage and upper body has been completed. It is useful where the client has shown signs of apnoea or shallow breathing, and brings them into a fuller capacity of their breathing, returning it to its natural power and rhythm. The apex of the lung reaches up into the shoulder girdle.

Stand behind at the head of the ZB table facing the client at a distance whereby you can use your whole body in the fulcrum. Curl both hands to form loose fists.

Gently place these at the top of the front of the client's rib cage, just beneath the clavicle and medial to the coracoid process. Find a comfortable nestle on this area of the chest and pectoral muscle.

Then give the client the instruction to take a full breath up into where your hands are meeting them. When they reach a full inhalation, give them the instruction to breathe out and follow their chest, maintaining contact as they exhale. Calibrate the rhythm of this interaction once or twice so they know how you are requesting them to participate.

Then, as they inhale up into their upper chest, provide a working resistance with your hands whilst encouraging them to breathe fully. On each of the exhalations, follow them down, maintaining contact but without pressure.

Perform three or four repeated guided inhalations and exhalations. On the last working inhalation, whilst your hands are providing resistance to their breathing, gradually release your contact. They may momentarily pause in the fullness of their inhalation. Then give them the instruction to 'Breathe naturally', allowing them to enjoy its rhythm and power.

The momentary pause when you remove your hands can give a sense of expansion and being filled with the nourishment of breath that can be revelatory.

This fulcrum should be performed with care, working with the client in respecting the condition of their structure and energy. Using the gentle strength of your whole body coming from your lower centre of gravity helps in calibrating the level of your touch, and gives this fulcrum its power.

Earth element

Characteristic movement of qi: centred orientation.

Body correspondence: flesh, muscle and connective tissues.

Location: central region – the crossing of all four elements, a centred place from which they can all interact in harmony.

Season: late summer – when nature is bearing fruits, having reached a stage of maximum growth before the change of autumn.

Qi experience: being at home in self, calm, collected wellbeing, nourished by that which feeds you, for example nurturing touch, which you become yourself and in turn give back to care for others.

Virtue of Earth: ability to be in the centre and know all sides – to be able to relate to all directions/respond and nourish all sides from a centred axis – bringing about body-mind unity.

The earth of the Earth element is the soil, the ground from which comes the nourishment that constantly rebuilds our life and form. The earth in heaven/earth contains the elemental character for Earth but is distinct in character, referring to our planet in the relationship between heaven and earth. This double meaning of the same word also occurs in the English language.

The quality of the qi of Earth has a presence we can trust and rely on. In a Zero Balancing session this quality is there right after the client first lies down. This is sometimes introduced before the opening half moon vector.

Standing at the end of the ZB table by the client's feet, use the relaxed power of your whole body, simply press and hold their lower legs with gentle compression, affirming and contacting their bones. The touch gives confirmation of their structure and energy and brings their body-mind present prior to the opening half moon vector.

The Zero Balancing logo is of a simple lifting fulcrum. It is a memorable graphic symbol. In relation to the practice of Zero Balancing, all that it lacks is a base line underpinning it, indicating that a fulcrum is not 'in mid air' but is acting from a stable 'earth'.

Earth is at the centre of all the other four elements. The central region is a place, not a direction. It is at the crossing of all the four directions, receiving their influences, interacting with them and reconnecting with them for their replenishment. Being in the middle, it is able to take in the qi from all sides, actively relating to the four from a centred place.

The experience of the centre – in Chinese, *zhong* (中) – is of a place whereby the four are in good relations, bringing together by the nature of a centre emerging from a crossing of the four, incorporating the virtue of a well-placed fulcrum – in its stable constancy – allowing orientation according to whatever direction is needed.

A fulcrum in Zero Balancing has a stable point around which structure and energy can orient and balance. The nature of a fulcrum is that it comes from a place of rooted stability and is held in place, allowing balancing to happen around its central orientation.

An essential aspect of what makes a fulcrum effective is known in Chinese as *chang*, meaning 'the constant'. When a fulcrum has been built and is in place, it is essential it be held still, without wavering or wobbling. In the conversation between your structure and energy and the client's structure and energy, constancy allows them time and place to respond and rebalance, implicit in the invitation the fulcrum is offering. It requires a secure, well-earthed held point, and being open to the possibility of change.

Zero Balancing nurtures the ability to adapt. This essential response is integral to our wellbeing. It enhances our ability to respond to forces and stresses from every direction whilst knowing where we are at the centre, as a dynamic pivot as well as a still middle around which everything rotates.

A well-placed fulcrum can be instrumental in transformation occurring. In Chinese the character for transformation is *huà* (化), which has the etymology of a human being turning head over heels, reflecting a radical change in their state of being.

In Chinese medicine the organs associated with Earth are those of digestion. The stomach and spleen receive the food from all directions, transform it, and then return it by transporting it to the four quarters to nourish, renew and maintain our form.

The virtue of the qi of the centre is that its power has a gathering centrality essential in balancing as well as being able to 'hold things in place'. This is implicit in the nature of being in the centre. A weakening of the force of central gathering may lead to our structure and energy being able to 'keep things in place', whether that leads to prolapses or misalignments. Our form and posture as a biped means that our bodies need a distinct awareness of our centre of gravity to, for example, quadrupeds.

The ability of Earth to be in communication with the qi energy of the other four elements can be seen in the Chinese character *tong* (通), which has the meaning of free communication, having access throughout or penetrating without obstruction.

> *Tong bu Tong, Tong bu Tong. Where there is pain there is no free communication. Where there is free communication there is no pain.*

This is a well-known aphorism in Chinese that uses another character also Romanised as *tong* that has a different meaning of pain or soreness:

> *When the vital spirits thrive and the qi are not scattered, then there is perfect order (Li)*
> *Perfect order, then equilibrium (Jun)*
> *Equilibrium then free communication (Tong)*
> *Free communication (Tong), then the spirits (Shen)*
> *With the spirits*
> *There is nothing which is not seen,*
> *In listening there is nothing which is not heard,*
> *In doing there is nothing which is not accomplished,*
> *Thus worries and concerns cannot enter and perverse qi cannot strike.*
>
> (Huainanzi, Chapter 7 – Jing Shen, quoted in
> Bromley, Freeman and Hext 2010)

A good fulcrum brings the power of a central place of Earth and it being open to connection with all, orienting and transforming as required.

The qi of Earth is that the centre of qi incorporates and allows the ability to adapt to all movements of life's structural energetics. This virtue of adaptability is essential in maintaining our equilibrium with all the changes of living in the relative world.

In the movements of Taiji Quan there is a section of radical moves with the name 'Fair lady works the shuttles'. The practitioner moves and turns to face all four directions, rotating from a centred axis. Its title refers to the 'weaving maiden' sitting in a centred place at her spinning wheel with awareness of the four directions. This image is illustrated in the meditation diagram engraving at the white cloud monastery in Beijing, in the centre of the trunk of the body.

At the completion of Zero Balancing, following the closing half moon vector, the Zero Balancer crosses their forearms and holds the client's feet or ankles with their opposite hands. This contacts the bones of your body with a touch that gives a sense of conclusion to the session and the inner 'figure of eight' movement that confirms their structural energetic presence.

If, when standing, the person requires further confirmation, they may be asked to move in a staccato manner that engages both sets of limbs in a 'cross crawl' movement.

I close this piece on the Earth element and return to the meaning of the characters for Wu Xing mentioned in the section of this book introducing the five elements (see page 114). Walking is the perfect activity to integrate a Zero Balancing session. Moving the body including both arms and legs in a simple but complex crossing movement brings the five elements and inner centres of balance into integrated motion.

A SINGLE FINGER FULCRUM AT THE SCAPULA

The scapula is one of two bones of the shoulder girdle, a structure resting lightly on the upper trunk/overlying the thoracic cage and articulating in a shallow ball and socket joint with the humerus, the bone of the upper arm. This structure and joint together allow a wide range of movement. This freedom of movement and ability to stretch out our arms, touch others and embrace is a perfect place to recognise the manifestation of the rising, expansive energy of Fire.

The shoulder girdle is the structure that connects the trunk, especially the chest, with the arms and the arms with the trunk. The scapula is structurally energetically connected with the neck and thence to the head, brain and senses.

The shoulder girdle is made up of two freely moveable bones whose only bone articulation lies at the sternoclavicular joint. In good structural energetic health the shoulder girdle has a high degree of freedom in its movements.

When the arm is raised there is a natural movement in the scapula to accommodate the motion. For every ten degrees of arm motion there is an accompanying five degrees of scapular motion. In good health the 'mantle' of your shoulder girdle rests easily on your trunk. If your 'yoke is heavy, let your burden be light', as the saying goes.

In core Zero Balancing, the client's arm is moved through posterior circumduction and attention is given to the range and quality of movement in the shoulder joint as a way of appreciating the articulations of the ribs with the thoracic vertebrae.

It is also possible to use this movement to evaluate movements of the shoulder girdle. The second hand rests over the client's upper scapula and you can often also have contact with the clavicle.

Underneath the scapula is a 'breathing space' that, along with the muscle connections of the serratus anterior, relate the medial scapula with individual ribs.

There may be several places of tenderness on the body of the scapula that will benefit from touch. However, for this fulcrum it is valuable to locate the centre of the bone. What is the centre of a triangle?

Bring your hands under the client's body and locate the dimensions of the bone with your hands. Identify the horizontal 'spine' of the scapula towards its superior edge and also the medial edge of the scapula. Imagine a line from one edge of the bone to the middle of its opposite side. This helps you to arrive at the centre of its roughly triangular shape.

When you have located where you will site your fulcrum, rest the back of your hand, anchoring them on the ZB table. Using one or two fingers, go through the sequence of taking out any loose play, taking up the slack, and engage the bones of your fingers with the flat bone of the scapula. Hold this simple lifting fulcrum with constancy. You are balancing the centre of the triangle of the scapula.

As it is a bone that knows the mobility of easy movement, this temporary stabilisation can be an unusual experience. The client may drop into an altered state. Time may feel suspended. Holding a bone with such freedom at its centre provides a point of orientation around which it can re-establish ordered movement. When this fulcrum is held with constancy, watch for breath responses and possible apnoea as the client drops deeply into themselves.

The 'breathing space' under the scapula, known as the subscapular bursa, helps as a shock absorber or insulator from the stresses of the outside world. Any force coming into the body can be lessened in its impact by the resilience of the scapula. Otherwise these forces and influences become caught up in the tensions and rigidity of this area, going directly into the rib cage, potentially disturbing the functioning of the lung and heart. These organs may be protected by the rib cage, but restriction and stiffness leaves them open to the effect of stress.

The centre of the scapula happens to match with an acupuncture point, with a name translated as Heavenly Ancestor, Small Intestine 11. Zero Balancing is not acupressure. However, this is a place where bone is relatively close to the surface, so you can have a bone-to-bone connection with Zero Balancing.

The movement of heaven is circular, and this place can be related to the motion of the shoulder girdle as well as the meridian pathway that then goes on to the neck and head. The spherical form of our head is likened to the circular orbiting movements of heaven. The pathway goes on to have two subsequent points that have heaven in their names, 16 and 17.

The Ancestor in the point name relates to the title given to the power of qi in the chest and the heart and lung, known as ancestral qi.

My experience of the beneficial altered state arises from when Dr Fritz Smith introduced this fulcrum to me in the 1980s, which I can recall in my body-mind memory. The combination of feeling well rooted in myself whilst being in an expanded awareness is still with me.

A Review of the Body-Mind 'Signatures' of Elemental Qi

Water: Ability to drop into the interior to restore – all the blessings of being able to float and deeply relax, trusting water as our bones to support us in our core.

Fire: Joyful enthusiasm and elation – rising expansive movement and settled warm relations with others as well as with sense of self.

Wood: Release from frustration/restriction + events going to plan – whether it is smooth, unfolding progression or coordinated movement well rooted, sustainable and flexible because it is fulfilling the Water element.

Metal: Rhythm in harmony, both letting go as well as taking in, knowing what is of true value.

Earth: Ability to be centred whilst knowing all sides, adapting to all directions, responding and, in turn, nourishing all sides.

We live in a time when the evidence and stresses of global climate change are increasingly evident and the reduction in biodiversity a statistical fact. Knowing the structure and energy of the elements within informs us of their vital nature and the unity of life. Through cultivating the conscious touch of Zero Balancing within our bodies, we regain respect for our fellow beings and the planet that is our home.

14

Zero Balancing Touches the Body-Mind

I t is possible through Zero Balancing to bring a person into touch with hidden tensions they are holding and aid their release. Our body is a repository of our life's history. Whilst we may be aware or be reminded of a trauma we have experienced in our lives through bodywork, we may well be unconscious of what we are holding on to.

> If I have a thought, thought is a vibration – a thought wave. A group of thoughts becomes an idea, an idea a concept. A concept strongly held over time becomes a belief system, an article of faith. You identify with a held belief.
>
> All of us are dealing with our inheritance, beliefs, strategies from childhood, society, education, family, history, culture. We may take on a belief system that works at a certain time of life or in a certain situation. Then when we change and grow up this unconscious behaviour is deeply ingrained and we fail to adapt or change to new circumstances.
>
> We can hold beliefs in our body-mind as held tensions which we no longer need. We put energy into defending, maintaining or identifying with them.
>
> They are accessible through touch. Zero Balancing bodywork releases held vibration, releases a person in a non-verbal way through touch to allow them to be who they actually are, in the present. (Fritz Smith speaking in a workshop)

Beliefs from our early upbringing can imprint in the structural energetics of our body-mind. We may not realise the 'pressures of the past' we retain that unnecessarily distort our freedom to live in the present. We may still be holding the admonitions and instructions of early life in our body-mind. We may still be identifying with judgements and criticisms from when we were growing up that we identify with but that we no longer need to. Whilst these may have had their importance in our early lives, they can become inbuilt and be unconsciously restricting the way we are living now.

We may have a distorted sense of our body-mind form with varied levels of dysmorphia in our structural energetic awareness. Zero Balancing can be of value as a reality check, returning a person into touch with their real selves, transcending the ideas they hold of who they think they are.

Zero Balancing can also play an important role in relation to different stages in our lives. The transition between adolescence and adulthood can have its particular difficulties, as can that between active work and retirement. Zero Balancing can be beneficial in successfully traversing such key changes.

The possibilities of the benefits of Zero Balancing are still being explored in myriad applications. It has been taught to a wide range of healthcare professionals who are using it as a therapeutic approach in its own right, as well as in combination with their existing practice. The range of their professional training includes doctors, acupuncturists, massage therapists, chiropractors, osteopaths, counsellors, speech therapists and homeopaths.

It may be a popular notion to simply bracket Zero Balancing as only addressing musculoskeletal issues. However, its ability to touch a person's body-mind and for transformation on broader levels means that it should not be limited or its practice marginalised by narrow categorisation that reduces its potential.

15

Zero Balancing as a Bodywork Meditation

The beginning of a Zero Balancing workshop opens with a meditation. This has been integral to the process of learning of Zero Balancing since it was first taught.

To start with, you are often asked to sit forward on your seat, so that the bones of your ischium are in clear contact with the firmness of your chair. This chair–bone contact gives you a rooted connection reminiscent of the firm but gentle nature of Zero Balancing touch. The meditation may involve a guided journey through the body, or visualisations of fundamental structural energetic relationships.

It is possible for the practice of Zero Balancing to become a form of active bodywork meditation for its practitioners. It requires you to be fully present in your own structure and energy, with qualities of relaxed attention. It demands a level of interactive awareness and sensitivity that keeps you engaged, in the moment, and consciously in touch.

Meditation brings you congruent with the rhythm of your breath and being present in your body. Your attention returns to alignment and balanced contact with your inner centres.

Both meditation and Zero Balancing can quieten the chattering of the mind. They cultivate inner attention and an ability to not be unnecessarily disturbed by what is going on around you. I remember giving a Zero Balancing session where the noise of roadworks unexpectedly started up close by. I was concerned it would adversely affect my client. However, they told me at the end of the session that although they had been aware of the sound, it had not become an annoyance. The session had taken them deep inside themselves whereby other sounds did not disturb them.

The rhythm of evaluation, fulcrums and re-evaluation gives order and feedback to your investigative activity and the nature of your interaction. The protocol of core Zero Balancing provides a valuable structure, capable of adapting to the variety of individual needs.

The attention to the quality of touch brings you into your hands. Your whole body becomes engaged as Zero Balancing activates your own structure and energy with relaxed power and attention. This brings an ease into your activity so that it feels less like 'work' and more like a fascinating journey. When you are in touch with energy it can feel like being on a moving travelator, of the sort found at airports or some underground stations. The session then feels like it 'takes off' with a momentum of its own.

> Your touch gets wiser as you do. There is no end to the develop-ment and refinement that is possible as you learn to adapt to different people and situations. Learning Zero Balancing has similarities to learning Tai Ji Quan. The protocol is straight-forward, simplicity is what gives it its power. I recommend you have your mind quiet, allowing you to focus your attention on the client and your fingertips. The Zero Balancer get healthier by the practice of Zero Balancing, more centred, more spiritually awake. Why? Because every time you put in a fulcrum and hold it at a moment of stationary quietness, part of you goes into that condition and allows your true nature to manifest. (Dr Fritz Smith, teaching students at an osteopathic college in Tokyo, Japan, 1998)

The Zero Balancer pays attention to the client and their 'working signs' that indicate their response to the work. This gives important guidance to crafting the pace of a session, sensing when to pause and allowing them space, and when to bring the Zero Balancing to completion.

Working with the stages of engaging structure and energy, recognising the feel of the blue line in your hands, cultivates a growing awareness. This is capable of continuing refinement as you learn to adapt to a variety of people and become informed by experience. Zero Balancing gets you out of your head and into your hands without denying your intelligence.

It is important to give prospective clients an outline description of a session so that they are properly informed and agree to receive Zero Balancing. A session is very individual to that person and specific to them. Ideally clients come to Zero Balancing with open-minded curiosity rather than a multiplicity of expectations.

Responses to a session vary according to a variety of factors. A Zero Balancing session may be a restorative rest, helping clear the client of discomfort or inflexibility. It can take the client into deep relaxation, clearing levels of tensions they were unaware of holding but glad to be free of. It can be a rich remembering and body-mind confirmation of who they truly are. A session can realign them with their core and a sense of fundamental repair. Some Zero Balancing can leave clients profoundly touched and transformed.

One variable in the nature of this interaction is the level of attention of the Zero Balancer. The cultivation of awareness is aided by clarity in their own structure and energy. Meditation quietens the body-mind and centres consciousness in their being so that they are able to be present with the person.

Zero Balancing is a practice that works with inner principles and that has a built-in body-felt feedback. Principles are living tools that provide an essential guide and reality check. The feedback from working with inner principles develops the objective witness. The hallmarks of this are an embodied objectivity that is well grounded in a tangible reality of life. Its characteristics are impartiality, receptive and responsive to change, with a non-judgemental approach.

The Zero Balancer is 'working with' the client rather than 'doing something to them'. The practice requires the Zero Balancer to fully be with the client. As a practitioner, you may be aware of the beneficial altered states of consciousness that the client is having.

The interaction requires a level of attentiveness and awareness in which you, as the Zero Balancer, are completely present as the responsible guide.

The fulcrums and vectors have the nature of invitations to return to balance, rather than insistent demands or forced imposition to change. You are setting up the conditions whereby transformation can occur if the client takes up the invitation. This is another aspect of their active involvement, often at a level without words or conversation. It develops a practice that requires the Zero Balancer to be fully present with the client. You may become aware of your being in ways that transcend the limitations of your own 'identity'.

Fulcrums and vectors work within a normal range of motion and so have a safety and acceptability for the client. Their value is that they can beneficially affect the quality and range of movement in the end range of the motion of joints without specifically needing to work in the end range.

The clarity of touch through working at the interface maintains a working connection of distinction between the Zero Balancer and the client without a sense of separation. Zero Balancing uses the silence of touch to develop a non-verbal rapport.

The Zero Balancer is tuned with the dynamic of change, knowing and working in the relative world, whilst simultaneously being aware of that which is beyond change. The skill is being able to engage the person using fulcrums and vectors, held with stability and constancy, with openness to their potential. This complementary skill is there in the touch as well as the means of touching. The stable centre of a fulcrum combines stillness with the flexibility of its axis allowing orientation and rebalancing.

The practice and unfolding development for a Zero Balancer brings you into an awareness of the frontiers of your learning, and that which you may not yet have grasped or still awaits comprehension. Zero Balancing excites a natural attraction to continued growth in which learning can be a genuine exploratory adventure of discovery. There is a term in Zero Balancing known as 'growing edge'. It is where your understanding is stimulated and challenged by the practice of

Zero Balancing. Both the Zero Balancer and the client benefit from the perception of 'growing edge'.

> I put my fingers on their body with a fulcrum and wait until their body and the person's mind can let go. In yoga practice there is the experience of the frontier of new possibility that is the growing edge. This is there for the beginner as well as for the yogi. Everyone is doing it for the first time. In Zero Balancing we are asking them to run a risk. In many ways it is highly safe. They are lying on the ZB table in secure circumstances and you are just touching them in a fairly non-invasive way, but you are offering them an experience of their growing edge and the territory beyond. The spin-off from a Zero Balancing session is that, having processed the risk here, they can then be ready to accept change in their life. (Dr Fritz Smith, teaching in a workshop)

Zero Balancing has attracted authentic seekers who want to learn a bodywork skill and art and, as with meditation, discover their own nature. The Chinese recognised that important skills, from calligraphy to medicine, embodied the discipline of self-reflective development. To practise on this level can be recognised as a path of authentic cultivation of being human.

The perception of the structure and energy of forms in Chinese can be seen in the character for this knowledge, *li* (理), which has the meaning of the internal pattern of life. The etymology of the character shows the 'veins' in jade that reveal its inner life and its character. *Li* is the intrinsic organisational pattern of structural energetic form. In our body *li* can be seen manifesting in the fibres in muscle or trabeculae in bone.

What is the *li* of a human being? What is its structure and energy? How do you access and work with the *li* of a living person with your hands?

We possess a vertebrate spine and stand upright on two legs. Our heels have developed their structure and energy in a form distinct to animals such as quadrupeds. They give us a specific sense of our standing in the world and relate contact with the earth with our brains and senses. Our hands have also developed particular abilities and sensitivities as we use them in combination with our brain and senses.

In relation to the acuity and breadth in some other creatures' senses, human beings are sometimes quite limited. We have developed machines to extend the range of our perceptions.

We know what happens when, for example, we are bed-ridden and how quickly we lose muscle tone and usage. If we no longer use senses, they, too, atrophy or we lose perceptive awareness.

In the range of our senses, those of eyesight and hearing have been explored and served by investigation. However, the sense of human touch has often been less appreciated or cultivated. This can be seen in the relative lack of publications that record and celebrate the explorations and discoveries of bodyworkers in this last century. The work of Ida Rolf, Moshé Feldenkrais, Milton Trager or John McTimoney, to name a few important pioneers, has received insufficient attention. Dr Fritz Smith has made a unique contribution to the bodywork world, developing awareness of conscious human touch within the vehicle of an approach that is accessible and applicable and particularly relevant to our contemporary lives.

Touching our bones touches the core essence of our structure and energy. Zero Balancing touches our tangible living inner form and the vitality of space we inhabit. It does so in ways that are respectful and meaningful. It reconnects a person with their *li*. It becomes manifest, aligned and harmonised.

Seeing and experiencing Fritz Zero Balance people can feel like being sculpted. However, this is not imposing his idea of how the person should be upon them. It is more like a sculptor who reveals the intrinsic nature of the material they are working with. Touching bone with firm, clear gentleness goes through the surface, through the cosmetic cover to the core of the person, a core that we are often unaware of.

It is working in ways that reveal the essential 'grain' of a person's living form. In Daoism this is often expressed as the simplicity of the 'uncarved block' or 'unbleached silk', the unadulterated nature of who the person really is, beyond their identifications, ideas or attachments.

In the writings of the Chinese philosopher Zhuang Zi, he refers to the story of a butcher named Ding who developed considerable skills. Ding used his knife to carve with effortless ease and skilful accuracy, without the blade ever becoming blunt. He knew how to cut following the seam and particularly working in the spaces between the muscles, the openings and energy of the body.

These are skills arising from internal stillness, pure attention, getting out of the way, touch that carefully listens and resonance with what is being worked with. This sensitivity manifests from cultivating an inner quietude that awakens a clarity and openness in our mind and body.

It is possible to be in touch with the tangible and the intangible, form and space, inner and outer, back and front, subtle and substantial, structure and energy, all simultaneously, the universal manifesting within the individual, the relative and that which is unchanging.

> *A human being follows the ways of earth,*
> *The earth follows the ways of heaven,*
> *Heaven follows the ways of the Dao,*
> *The Dao follows that which is naturally so.*
>
> (Daodejing, *Chapter 25*)

Holding the Two as One

Consciousness moves in jumps – two to one to zero.

A Zero Balancer introduces a vector, holding the person's two ankles in gentle half moon with dorsiflexion. Holding the person's legs with equal engagement, there are times when the person may experience a profound response of an awareness of a central flow through their entire body. The two legs are being held, the curves of their spine relax, and the unity of their spine is activated all the way up to their head.

This 'opening' can feel both expansive whilst being held within the person's body, but not in any 'restricted' way. This is a body-felt sense of unity with a complementary awareness.

When two complementary aspects are brought together and held in equanimity, there is a potential for change and transformation to occur. If the two are apparent opposites, bringing them into such relationship has particular potential.

What happens, for example, in humour? A joke can often be two pieces of information that cannot be held together in our minds at the same time. They may be contradictory or incompatible. When they are presented together the mind is challenged and, unable to hold this, erupts into a laugh as a release to our body-mind. It jumps us beyond our previous state of mind.

A verbal pun is a simple example of similar-sounding words that can have two different and sometimes opposing meanings. For example, a bookseller in England was mistakenly asked for a copy of George Orwell's book *Dining Out in Paris and London*!

The tension in the mind of holding both is diffused with a laugh or, in the case of a pun, sometimes a groan, as the play on words is realised.

Visual illusions can be of an image with two different possible levels of interpretation. There is a well-known one that is either the outline of a vase or two heads in profile facing each other. What happens if you are able to keep both interpretations of the one image active simultaneously?

The skill of seeing a 'hidden' image in a visual graphic is used in the insignia for FedEx. Are you able to perceive the arrow within the colour and space of their sign?

Interpreting a 'magic eye' stereo image requires you to relax your eye muscles and any tension of trying to see. When you are able to let go, it is possible for the apparent three images to appear and you can 'interpret it' from the jumble of visual information on the page.

Zen practice uses the challenge of the *koan*, an apparently impossible question posed to the novice to answer. If an attempt is made to answer with normal 'intellect', then the mind can get caught up in impossible contradiction. If it is 'held' in the novice's body-mind, it can trigger a jump into the zero reality of no-mind. The challenge to our normal ways of thinking can become jumps of insight and revelation.

What is happening in our perceptions? Are there commonalities in this phenomenon when this happens across different senses? Can this occur through touch?

In Zero Balancing it is possible to give the person two different sensory inputs at the same time. They may interpret these as contradictory. For example, when holding a fulcrum, they cannot distinguish between the strength of your touching them and the pressure of their own body. Or holding a fulcrum that combines both stillness and movement. The fundamental pairing of holding structure and energy simultaneously in Zero Balancing is an example of such integral pairing.

The body-mind can become challenged by having two contrary or opposite sensations or inputs being introduced to it simultaneously. Sometimes the touch in Zero Balancing may be one of both pleasure and on the edge of discomfort. In terms of where you are in the diagram of touching structure and energy, these are fulcrums at the far right end of the box. The person is still responding rather than in reaction, and you are still 'in the box'.

The person's body-mind can find it unable to hold this double sensation and can jump into new levels of awareness that are recognised as beneficial altered states of consciousness. These happen in conditions of safety within a session. They are body-felt, so can be integrated by the person. They are not being forced on the person but arise as part of the interactive working relationship between the Zero Balancer and the client.

Bringing two aspects into balance can instil a new sense of equilibrium and degrees of being in harmony.

What is described above is, however, much more than this. What is being described is above and beyond that level of perception. It is an understanding of what happens when you are able to hold the apparent paradox of both interpretations at the same time.

It is an appreciation of the way beneficial altered states of consciousness can be triggered. A Zero Balancing fulcrum becomes a catalyst for an internal jump in the person's awareness.

Knowing how to touch in such a fine-tuned way is a key development in the skill of Zero Balancing. An essential aspect of this skill is being able to hold the two with interface touch. This is an important condition in aiding the catalyst of change to take place and 'precipitate' a jump in the person's consciousness. As this happens in the context of a Zero Balancing bodywork session, it has safety as well as the opportunity for change to be integrated as a beneficial embodied experience.

Such altered states are recognised by, for example, perceptions of a different awareness of the duration of time or of space to those a person is familiar with. You are fully alive in your body with awareness of relaxed flexibility. There can be a sense of expansion whilst being fully present in yourself, Zero Balanced.

The Relative and Unchanging

Zero Balancing enhances our ability to live in the relative world by reminding our body-mind of its intrinsic ability to adapt to change and know balance. The skill of harmonising with fundamental rhythms is cultivated by engaging the structure and energy with the internal pivot of fulcrums. These provide an essential awareness of centre, nurturing instinctive orientation.

Zero Balancing can also bring you into awareness beyond the everyday parameters of relativity, beyond the world of change. (This is explored further in the sections in this chapter on 'Holding the Two as One' and The 'Manifesting and the Return').

Zero Balancing balances fundamental alignments with the structure and energy of your foundation and semi-foundation joints and their interrelationships. It brings you into wider alignment by orienting you to forces beyond your form.

The two functions of the energetics of our body are to connect the individual to the greater whole of nature whilst enabling them to function as an autonomous being.

This fundamental skill is nurtured in Zero Balancing by returning a person to a body-felt sense of flexibility. In a larger sense it assists in being able to adapt to where you are in time and space, whilst being more fully present in yourself.

The development of the awareness of both is of value to any therapist. The skill of a Zero Balancer is to know and be able to hold both simultaneously, whilst staying present and being of service to the client. The Zero Balancer has a clear sense of the beginning, middle and end of the session.

The importance of engaging, holding fulcrums and taking hands in an appropriate rhythm for that person is an essential skill. Interface touch lets them know who they are and who you are, lessening projection and potential confusion.

Zero Balancing sessions are held without any accompanying music. This can become a distractive intrusion, entraining them to external rhythms rather than those integral to who they are.

Generally unnecessary conversation is minimised as it can distract the client from returning to the quietude of their interior.

At the end of a session it is important to respect how the client is. After the Zero Balancer has completed and is no longer in direct touch, the process of balancing may well continue. It is important to respect what is happening within the person and the silence of this moment.

The client may be in a heightened wordless state. They may be in an 'expanded' state of sensitivity. What is said to them can easily imprint or have greater significance than the Zero Balancer may realise.

There may be a temptation to talk to them about what you found, as if you were diagnosing their condition. It is important to recognise that they are very likely in a process of change, and what you have felt or discovered may well be in process and have moved on.

What you say may reinforce previous patterns rather than affirm changes. Generally it is better to confirm what you found that was positive, or say very little.

If they appear to be in an altered state, make sure they are aware of the real world. Sometimes they may be asked to make movements known as cross crawl, moving their arms and legs in a staccato action. As required, make sure they are wearing clothing that keeps them suitably warm. Encourage them to walk around in nature and to have something to eat, or rest as required.

Essences are everywhere because they rebuild bone marrow and the brain in the skull. We understand the quality of the essences and the force with which they are assimilated, incorporated and maintained is the condition of the bones or the marrow, or the accuracy of the mind in the brain and so on. When the essences (jing) are good they are able to welcome the presence of the spirits (shen) and to support the enlightenment coming from the spirits. This is also called jingshen. (Rochat de la Vallée, *Essence, Spirit, Blood and Qi*, 1999, p.35)

Centre

One of the four Confucian classics has the name *Zhong Yong*. Its title has been variously translated as *The Doctrine of the Mean*, *Central Harmony*, *The Invariable Middle* or *The Unwobbling Pivot*. The *yong* has the meaning of everyday use – ordinary, common and fundamental. *Yong* puts the principle of centrality into normal life, as an essential human awareness. The classic expounds its human and social importance. *Zhong* is that which never deviates, that which never changes. What never changes is the continuity of change.

It is so essential and common that it is hidden and we become unconscious of it. There is nothing more perceptible than that which is hidden. Water similarly is so universal and forms the largest part of our body that we forget about it. We similarly forget about the air we breathe that is essential for our life, until it becomes scarce or polluted.

Zero Balancing embodies the experience of *Zhong Yong* as a living awareness. This is so in the practice of Zero Balancing as well as being nurtured within the client. The centre unites a person with themselves as well as their vital relationship with heaven and earth.

It has a normality, rightness and commonness, embodied common sense, whilst simultaneously being something extraordinary, beyond words. It awakens in the receiver and the Zero Balancer a living interconnected uprightness of interrelationship, reflecting what heaven has bestowed upon us: the human nature that is heaven within us living on this planet.

Bodywork that really touches a person can sometimes give access to hidden emotion that wells up during a session. Emotions may be held in soft tissue so that it is a more common experience during deep tissue work. Bone that is the focus of touch in Zero Balancing 'holds' a deeper level of issues and may be less likely to result in emotion release. This has also been my experience of Zero Balancing. During a session a client may shed a tear or laugh or chuckle as they just 'got' a joke, but emotional catharsis is rare. However, emotions are neither ignored nor denied. In Zero Balancing, a person is simply held whilst they go through the rapids of any turbulence or release.

In the early sections of the *Zhong Yong* there is a passage:

> Before the emotions of pleasure, anger, sorrow and joy are awakened the state is called centrality (Zhong). When these emotions are aroused and each and all attain measure and degree, it is called harmony. The state of centrality is the great root of the world and harmony is its universal path. Let centrality and harmony be realised to perfection and a happy order will prevail throughout heaven and earth and all things will be nourished and flourish. (*Zhong Yong*, Chapter 1, section 4)

The nature of centrality returns you to a place prior to the arising of emotions.

Zhong is the ability to know both sides, being in the world and being able to work with awareness at the origin of left and right, the centre. This leads to another level of integration, unification and communication, working with and knowing the two as well as knowing the source from which the two arise.

The *Zhong Yong* is sometimes regarded as being mystical, but it has down to earth meaning for everyday awareness. If you replace *Zhong* with *Dao* you get a sense of its mystery. The centre is the midpoint between the manifest and the un-manifest – the source of manifestation. Zero Balancing can reconnect us with the origin. As Zero Balancing is a non-verbal therapy, this can take us into what is beyond words. This awareness of the *Dao* is expounded in the first chapter of *Daodejing* – the *Dao* that can be spoken of is not the whole *Dao*. When you start talking about it, you may have gone away from being in it. If it is the nature of life, it is not possible to be without it for a moment.

The centre is, in fact, not a place or an area, but the ability to interact to distinguish and respond as required from awareness beyond the two. The centre is not a thing, but the ability to know and hold apparent paradox and allow the opportunity for transcendence.

We live in a body that has many paired structures and functions – two legs and arms, two hands and feet, two kidneys and lungs, two lungs, two eyes, ears, nostrils, two hemispheres of brain, rhythms of inhalation and exhalation, ingestion and elimination, etc. We need to know the two in their paired activity and being in good harmony of their interrelationship, whilst also knowing what is between and beyond the two.

Master Cheng Man-ch'ing wrote an essay on the vital importance of *Zhong* in relation to Taiji Quan:

> Taiji, the yin/yang symbol, manifests the change and trans-formation of all the myriad creatures on earth. Zhong Yong examines this change and attains a state of non-inclination and changelessness – it possesses the principle of constancy. To understand Taiji but not Zhong Yong is to lose the applicability of yin/yang transformation; to understand Zhong Yong but not Taiji is to lose the steady axis. Taiji is the balance beam. Zhong Yong is the pivot point. (From the introduction to Professor Cheng's commentary on the *Zhong Yong* in Man-ch'ing 1997)

If I place myself in the centre in the five elements, where is it? It is at the intersection of the lines that cross and connect to the other four elements, four directions and four seasons. The centre is implicit in the five elements. The designation of Earth being in the centre is not an area but the ability to bring together, transforming in order to be redistributed. *Zhong* is an activity of equilibrium, being neither north nor south, east nor west, left nor right, up nor down, inside nor outside. Equilibrium is the virtue of the centre.

Zero Balancing is more than just equalising things out. It is about bringing alive that which allows balancing to occur of itself, reconnecting a person to the very source of equilibrium.

The Manifesting and the Return

The myriad beings flourish together, I simply contemplate their
return. For flourishing as they do each of them will return to their
origin. To return to its origin is to find peace. To find peace is to fulfil
one's destiny. To return to one's destiny is to be constant. To know
the constant is called illumination. (*Daodejing*, Chapter 16)

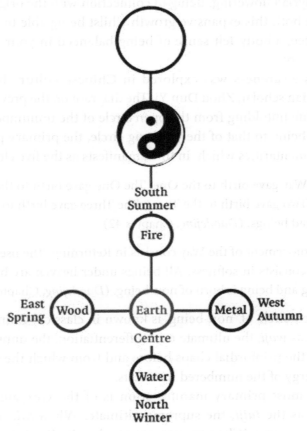

Wuji/taiji/the five elements

A Zero Balancing session may take a client into beneficial altered
states of consciousness. Fulcrums offer an invitation to orient in a
new level of balance. Transformation can occur if the person accepts
the invitation and is at a stage they are ready to change. All this

occurs in the safety of being in a relaxed, comfortable place on a ZB table. The Zero Balancer is an attentive guide, fully present, being there with the client. When Zero Balancing becomes truly meditative bodywork, the Zero Balancer can hold the middle point between the world in expansive growth and being present as the client reassembles and returns.

Zero is a place of origin. You can be aware of the life manifestation in its myriad flowering. Being in connection with the origin means you see both this expansive growth whilst being able to return to its source, a body-felt sense of being balanced in your structure and energy.

This awareness was explored in Chinese culture by a neo-Confucian scholar, Zhou Dun Yi. The diagram on the previous page shows life unfolding from the open circle of the unnumbered state of non-being to that of the yin-yang circle, the primary pairing of complementarities which, in turn, manifests as the five elements.

> The Way gave birth to the One. The One gave birth to the Two. The Two gave birth to the Three. The Three gave birth to all the myriad beings. (*Daodejing*, Chapter 42)

> The movement of the Way consists in Returning. The use of the way consists in softness. All beings under heaven are born of being and being is born of non-being. (*Daodejing*, Chapter 40)

The open circle of 'non-being' is known in classical Chinese or in Qigong as *wuji*, the ultimate non-differentiation, the unnumbered. *Wuji* is the primordial chaos before and from which the structure and energy of the numbered manifests.

The most primary manifestation is of the yin/yang pairing known as the *taiji*, the supreme ultimate. When *taiji* moves, it generates yang. When movement reaches its limit, it becomes tranquil. Through tranquillity the supreme ultimate generates yin. So movement and tranquillity alternate, becoming the root of each other, giving rise to the distinction of yin/yang.

By the transformation of yang and its union with yin, the five elements appear as Water, Fire, Wood, Metal and Earth, in harmonious order.

The interaction of these two forces engenders and transforms the myriad beings. The myriad beings produce and reproduce, resulting in unending transformation.

> The myriad beings returning lead to the Three. The Three to the Two. The Two to the One. The One to the Way of Transcendence. (From a commentary on the *Huang Ting Jing*, the *Yellow Court Classic*)

In returning, the five returns to the two, the two to the one and the one to the undifferentiated source – zero.

This is not merely some theoretical process but can be recognised in our body. The bones in our limbs follow a similar rhythm of manifestation, one to two to five. The upper limbs begin with the single bones of the humerus and femur, followed by the joints of the elbows and knees, then the paired bones of the radius and ulna, tibia and fibula and then the wrist and ankle, with the five metacarpals and metatarsals flowering into the five fingers and toes. This remembers the original budding of limb development in our foetal formation.

The Zero Balancer can hold a fulcrum encouraging reconnection with this unfolding as well as it being a recall, returning us to our origin, a reconnection with restoration and renewal.

Balancing structure and energy can give an awareness of centred equilibrium. This is not merely something 'induced' in the person; it is more a reminder of an inner orientation, an inner homeostatic functioning. This is a valuable harmonisation of levels of qi in a person's energy and structure that can enhance health and wellbeing.

Zero Balancing connects a person with the structure and energy of their bones, providing a fundamental rooting in their core structure. With this rooting in the substantial, subtle energies can be attracted to dwell and reside within the person.

Subtle energies would be recognised in Chinese as the energy of heaven, known as the *shen* spirits (Shen, 精神). The left part of this character shows the light shining down upon us from the sun, moon and stars by which heaven reveals its transcendent nature. The right-hand side of the character, in its ancient form showed two hands stretching a rope, with the larger meaning of expansion. In the evolution of the character, the rope became a man as a vertical stroke, with both hands girding his body with a sash.

The combination of both sides of the character gives a meaning of inviting and drawing down spiritual influx. Its nature potentially gives a sense of expansive revelation.

The definition of the *shen* spirits is found in the Chinese classics of *I Jing*, the *Book of Changes*, as well as in *Nei Jing*, the *Classic of Inner Medicine*.

> What Yin/Yang cannot probe, this is the spirits. (*Su Wen*, Chapter 66)

The spirits are beyond the differentiation of the two. You know their nature because they are incapable of being analysed. This is unity beyond any divisibility. They are not composed of yin/yang and therefore they are beyond any dualistic separation. Because of this they can ensure the movement and transformation that is human life. The spirits operate through their connection with the original mystery. They represent the original undifferentiated fusion in each person.

> It was in the USA at a conference with Fritz Smith. I lay down and he made a tour of my body with his hands. When I rose up I felt ten times higher than people around me, like Lilliputians. 'How long might this state of beatitude last?' I asked Fritz. He replied for a while and it lasted throughout the night.
>
> Several years later I had had a gentle stroke in my brain and I had difficulty moving and going quickly. I could not press my step. I then saw Fritz. He made the same circular touch. My face was radiant with joy and I was out of my wits with a sense of joy that made me feel like dancing.
>
> The third Zero Balancing was when we were together in Columbia with Ivan Illich after I had lectured. I found it very relaxing, without the elation. The surprise previously was that I felt younger.
>
> It is a valuable technique as it is working at the highest level of working on the spirits within the body. It is truly something. (Claude Larre, speaking of his experience of Zero Balancing)

16

The Relevance and Benefits of Zero Balancing

Regular Zero Balancing sessions release stress and tension held in our bodies and minds. It is the perfect therapy to maintain good health. It can relieve symptoms caused by energetic or structural imbalance through encouraging flexibility and alignment with an approach that is truly holistic. We recommend the client receives several sessions to begin with, then they should discuss with their Zero Balancer how they might continue the value of its benefits.

When Might You Consider Having a Zero Balancing Session?

Clearing stress and held tensions

Zero Balancing is perfect for when you feel your life is becoming overwhelmed by stresses you are struggling to deal with. These may be disturbing now, but ongoing disturbance may lead to imbalance and ill health. Clients frequently report feeling deeply relaxed and refreshed after a session, more able to adapt and deal with the causes of their stress. This leads to an improved capacity to enjoy a better experience of daily life:

> Zero Balancing has helped me deal with family crises and the unexplained pains and headaches I was suffering with. (Zero Balancing client)

Flexibility and posture

It is valuable to keep our body free of stiffness and to be well aligned. Zero Balancing enhances the quality of and range of motion in our joints. It helps the coordinated movement of our body. Zero Balancing is also a perfect bodywork therapy if you are practising yoga or Taiji, for example, as it works with similar principles of body-mind awareness:

> I feel taller and freer in my body. (Zero Balancing client)

Easing aches and pains

Body pain can occur where energy flow through our body becomes restricted, blocked or weakened, which can occur in areas of tension or overuse. By aligning the densest tissues of the bones and joints with the energy flowing through them, Zero Balancing facilitates the dissolution of limiting and uncomfortable patterns, thereby releasing energy back into them. As it touches both body and mind, it can ease discomfort arising from distress on many levels, clearing, calming and nurturing an experience of peaceful harmony within yourself:

> Zero Balancing has really helped clear the stiffness in my back which I had noticed since I've been carrying my new-born child. (Zero Balancing client)

Returning to being here and fully present

The constant overstimulation of electronic media can override our instincts for our true needs by seducing us into an over-activity that captivates our senses. Our awareness can become set on a level of 24/7 heightened alertness. The ability to know how to be at rest whilst being awake becomes lost. This may lead to disturbance in sleep patterns or background agitation that can precede exhaustion. Zero Balancing is a perfect way of bringing you back to yourself. It returns you to a real-time awareness of being back in touch with your real self through direct body-felt experience. An example of a modern challenge is recovering from jet lag. Your physical body has arrived, but you are left waiting for your energy and body rhythms to catch up. Zero Balancing is excellent at bringing your structure and energy congruent to clear the disruption of this dislocation:

> I feel I've returned home. (Zero Balancing client)

Problem solving and creative insights

It is frequently acknowledged that our perception of apparently insoluble situations or creative blocks can radically change when we gain access to deep levels of integration and rest within our minds and bodies. Managers and businesspeople, as well as artists, from composers to dancers, have found Zero Balancing valuable in the discovery of new solutions, or aiding a return to the creative flow of inspiration. As Zero Balancing addresses the whole body, it helps the realisation and subsequent manifestation of beneficial change:

> I stood up after the session, went straight to the piano and played a new piece which I had been struggling to write. (A composer, following Zero Balancing)

Reparative touch

Our natural responses to being touched can become distorted by traumatic experiences of abuse or prolonged physical or emotional pain. Zero Balancing establishes a clear relationship of safety between the therapist and the client whereby the boundaries of touch and communication are distinct and non-intrusive. The safety of this respectful interconnection enables the client to reclaim their body and rediscover the positive nature of human touch that develops a trust which has become lost or damaged.

Adapting to transitions in your life

Major changes such as moving house, changing jobs, bereavement or difficulties in close relationships are times when we need to be in the best of form. Zero Balancing provides a perfect support by tuning your structure and energy to optimum functioning so you can take on challenges through being at ease in yourself:

> Zero Balancing grounds me when I am in turbulence. I find it very affirming. (Zero Balancing client)

The final transition in life is that of the journey towards our passing. Several clients have come to me in the later stages of their life for bodywork. Zero Balancing has a place in hospice care alongside other therapeutic support. These clients have told me that they have richly appreciated the combination of non-verbal clearing of their past and being brought back to themselves. They feel wholly here and alive whilst being prepared for their departure.

17

The Value of Learning Zero Balancing for Acupuncture Practitioners

I started studying Zero Balancing four years after beginning practising traditional acupuncture. It soon became an essential source of insights. Zero Balancing complements my work with needles as well as giving me another therapeutic skill as they work wonderfully together. They could have been made for each other.

The benefits I have gained are manifold, so here I highlight a selection I have found particularly valuable.

Examining Skills

Zero Balancing is an aid to understanding the patient through touch. It supports the information from other ways of examining a person. Touching their structure and energy brings you into direct contact with the history stored in their bodies. I use my hands to interact with them and they have a direct non-verbal experience of the quality of how I will care for them. It aids gathering essential information about their overall condition as well as specific parts of their body that need attention. It teaches a number of skills common to practising and will enhance your acupuncture, even if you never practise Zero Balancing at all.

Developing Rapport

The quality of touching structure and energy not only reveals information but also equally importantly begins the process whereby you reassure the patient and gain their trust. By establishing a clear working relationship through conscious touch, you develop an effective patient–practitioner relationship. They relax and open up. Touch gives a direct empathy such that they are more likely to share the bigger picture, which may be critical in understanding how they are now and how best to serve them.

Preparation for Needling

Through the nature of how you touch them, the patient relaxes and there is an increase in their receptiveness to your treatment. Many acupuncturists have said that they only began to feel and realise what qi is when they studied Zero Balancing. It develops greater sensitivity to the way to find points, work and engage with qi and use needles most effectively.

Assessing Responsiveness to Treatment

Zero Balancing pays attention to how the patient responds to therapeutic intervention. It develops a keen awareness that guides your choice and quantity of treatment. As Dr Fritz Smith was developing Zero Balancing during his acupuncture studies, the two approaches are mutually sympathetic. I find I am more able to use acupuncture as a true art rather than practise it mechanically. It helps me realise acupuncture as a process of transformation rather than repetitive treatment.

Therapeutic Relationship

Zero Balancing develops a way of practice that works with the patient, rather than one of 'doing something to them'. This helps their involvement in the treatment. Traditional acupuncture usually addresses the roots of a person. It can be enormously valuable, for example after needling, to aid the larger integration of the treatment with a Zero Balancing.

The Value for the Practitioner

Through Zero Balancing I find I am more enlivened by being in practice, far less drained by the work and my own health has improved. My sensitivity and insight has significantly increased into how best to understand and treat patients more effectively.

> The wise behave in accordance with yinyang. The muscular forces and the network of animation are composed of a single qi, bones and marrow are strengthened, qi and blood flow one with another in a concerted movement. This being so, the result is the harmonious balance of the interior and exterior; the perverse influences cannot cause any harm; hearing and sight are acute. The qi is established in its perfection. (*Su Wen*, Chapter 3)

18

Zero Balancing – Building Bridges

> If you know structure, discover energy. If you know energy, discover structure. And with Zero Balancing, discover how to work with them together. (Dr Fritz Smith's invitation to practitioners of different healthcare approaches)

From early on in Dr Fritz Smith's teaching he saw the value and importance of bridging the worlds of established medicine and the world of alternative health so that they might inform each other for their mutual benefit. Zero Balancing has played an important role in bringing a wide range of therapists together to learn and exchange, with the bodywork providing the vehicle for a forum for cross-disciplinary interaction.

One of my first meetings with Fritz was at a seminar he had organised in California for a variety of medical specialists to give presentations to inform alternative healthcare practitioners. He entitled his first book *Inner Bridges* (1986). This documented his explorations and insights into what was known as the energy medicine. Fritz had the rigour and discipline of training and practice in Osteopathy and Medicine. He was aware of the clinical value of other therapeutic approaches, especially those rooted in Oriental traditions and bridging Western and Eastern wisdom.

The context of the times was such that significant acupuncture professionals such as Miriam Lee were being arrested for practising.

Legal and political conflicts were happening with ramifications for medicine. California was the first State to give acupuncture statutory recognition, and Fritz became the first MD to become licensed to practise acupuncture.

Zero Balancing incorporates many fundamental skills of a high-level therapeutic practice, which are common to many therapies.

This chapter explores some of the ramifications of this aspect of Zero Balancing. It can be taught as a bodywork approach in its own right and has been developed as a stand-alone therapy. It can also be used very successfully in combination with other healthcare professions. Zero Balancing teaches skills of touch sensitivity and understanding, applicable in many disciplines. Participants literally 'get it in their hands' as a means of directly embodied comprehension.

All too frequently, unfortunately, the practice of healthcare can exhaust its practitioners. This may be from being in contact with people in need in states of disorder or because of the intensity and quantity of work. However, this doesn't have to be so. It is possible to practise in ways that engage the practitioner, that attend to and serve the patient, whilst not deteriorating the health of the health worker. There is enormous value in using one's hands to listen to the patient's body. Such touch can help them 'feel heard', developing rapport and trust that may elicit information essential to a fuller understanding from the client. Zero Balancing enhances the healing relationship, benefiting both parties and assisting the active participation of the person in their health. Medical practice is increasingly without direct touch or contact, with the patient–practitioner dialogue being conducted via computer screens. The fundamental nature of the therapeutic relationship is changing, with hands-on contact becoming less common.

In this chapter I explore and make explicit some of the aspects that the discipline of Zero Balancing develops in relation to one of its original visions of building bridges. The workshops as well as the sessions function on multiple levels. Rather than providing a selection of 'fix-it' techniques, a Zero Balancing workshop holds the potential of whole other dimensions. It offers an invitation to the therapist to awaken their attention, using bodywork as the vehicle of comprehension, regardless of the particular therapy they practise.

Zero Balancing activates the structure and energy of the client in ways that mean they are participating through touch during the session. It develops an approach that initiates and invites the client's involvement, in a non-verbal manner, and at levels they may not be immediately aware of. It is very much more 'working with' compared to only 'doing to' or having a technique imposed on them.

Zero Balancing is a gentle approach that enables a person's own healing, activating its inherent intelligence. The nature and means by which this happens can vary. Different therapies use their own specific 'triggers' with an awareness of the sensitivity of the clients or patients. They may know from experience that a smaller dosage than normal of a medication works better for them. Some people are highly responsive. More is not better. The trigger may be minimal, with the person responding positively to a distant hint in measurable terms. Zero Balancing modulates the level of touch according to the area being worked, the person and the manner of their response.

Zero Balancing attracts levels of conscious attention from the Zero Balancer that requires them to be present, relaxed and awake in a session. They are sensitive to the interaction and to recognising the responses of the client. Such attentive monitoring contributes to the high degree of safety of its practice.

The Zero Balancer is aware of where they are touching whilst sensing wider responses and interconnections. It encourages awareness for both the client and practitioner. This perception pays attention to the context of wider interrelationships, such as to the other end or the other side or what is above and below, in relation to where they are working. Examples of other paired couples are back/front, left/right or interior/surface. I have written earlier about how an awareness of different levels of qi energy (such as two or three or five) can provide a way to develop a whole-istic vision and discern unity/disunity, wholeness or disconnection.

Levels of working are not hierarchical. Working directly on an area that the client is aware of being painful is often appropriate and has obvious relevance for them. Such work is not in contradiction with addressing the larger context. Whatever level or detail Zero Balancing addresses, it is always integrated through a whole session. This gives a completeness that brings local work to any area into context, allowing it to be easily recognised by the client and fully confirmed in their body-mind.

This is an example of an alternative therapy recognising and addressing the roots of imbalance. Another case would be in five-element acupuncture where an element or its relationships may be the underlying root of symptoms or disturbances. In Zero Balancing, the roots are addressed through balancing the foundation and semi-foundation joints, which a person may be oblivious of in relation to how they experience their functioning.

The development of a healthcare practitioner requires an awareness of different ways of perception that are complementary – analytical and analogical. Both need to be properly developed individually and honed with critical rigour through self-reflective application. The skill of a good therapist is to know both approaches and to be able to use and draw on the information and insight that both give. When these are well established and you are able to work with them in combination with accuracy, a new level of perception manifests.

A third level manifests that might be called empathetical perception. This can reveal itself in what may appear as intuitive insights, having an integral compassion towards those seeking care.

The analytical mode of thinking understands the world through dividing and separating in order to distinguish what is going on, and identify and label phenomena. It is the mode that is inbuilt in our Western education and science that we take without questioning its limitations. If you cannot measure or quantify what is happening, you may have reached the limits of being able to comprehend it. In medicine it is applied in differential diagnosis, which uses a systematic process of defining what is happening in a disease.

Analogical thinking is an integral aspect in traditional Chinese medicine. It looks at the patterns of what is happening, perceiving relationships and similarities in resonant character manifesting across different sensory data. It is useful in looking beyond the symptomatology to the root imbalance that may underlie the presenting problems. In five-element acupuncture a picture of what is happening involves the quality of qi with which the person describes their condition – their odour, colour and emotional expression. The data not only covers quantity, but also pays attention to quality. The Chinese classic of the pulse, *Mai Jing*, recognises 28 identifiable pulse qualities, although distinguishing eight is generally used in practice.

The perception is of the world in resonant vibration, yielding multiple patterns of related information. This observation of the world in classical China arises from what is known as Gan Ying, sometimes translated as 'Call and Response'. It is described in Chapter 6 of the *Huainanzi* classic. A note is played on a lute in one room and another lute in a separate room resonates sympathetically, without any action.

The observation of phenomena across the senses that arises from these insights is the basis of the resonant associations in Chinese classical medicine. An element shares a distinct but common energetic characteristic perceptible in a patient's colour, odour, sound of their voice and emotional expression.

The development of this sensory acuity requires a different approach and cultivation to that of analysis. It occurs when you are internally quiet, attuned and receptively open. It has an equal rigour in theory and practice to that of analysis, but requires a distinct development in its practitioners. It opens you to a world of understanding phenomena through interrelationships, patterns and rhythms, by appreciating the nature of the quality of qi energy.

It has been entitled 'correlative thinking' by A.C. Graham. Joseph Needham, the biologist and scholar of *Science and Civilisation in China* (1962), described its investigative approach as proto-scientific.

In our culture we use a knife and fork to eat our food. The knife cuts up the food, dividing it into edible portions, and the fork stabs or scoops it to transport it to our mouths. In the Orient chopsticks are used to eat. One stick is held relatively stable whilst the other is in relative movement to pick up food. In the Orient people hold one piece of food with the two, whilst in the West we cut, divide and stab. I use this as an example of our cultural differences and ways of perceiving and working with the world. Both are valid and can be used in combination.

In medicine, analysis (quantitative measurement) of, for example, blood tests, MRI scans or X-rays is used for information on which to base clinical judgements. However, borderline blood results – or scans – see inside but, for example, may show the structure is fine but the person is in real pain; they may show severe structural misalignment yet the person is not in significant discomfort.

It is important to recognise that all logics and approaches have their limitations, and it is essential to recognise when they are no longer being useful or are becoming a concept of reality, a belief system rather than a way that reveals insights.

Empathetical awareness appears when both analytical and analogical logic are alive and used in combination. Its characteristics are of insightful perceptions, from being able to see the wider picture, a natural compassion and a non-judgemental ability.

Our observation of the world since the Renaissance has implicitly involved perspective, even if we are unaware of this. Perspective, originally developed for military purposes, was utilised in architecture and in the visual arts. The hidden consequences of it are that it separates the seer from what is being seen, with their vision being taken from a single viewpoint. This externalises them as an outside observer and limits their view in time and space. The artist David Hockney made an insightful video taking us through a journey in two Chinese scrolls that recorded the Emperor's travels, one before the influence of perspective and the other following its introduction. The second revealed a distinct loss of richness in content as pre-perspective you could 'see around corners' and there was considerably less characterisation of people. Twentieth-century science has raised questions about the observer in relation to what was being observed and the potential influence affecting the accuracy of the observations. Zero Balancing recognises the cultivation of the objective witness, whereby analytical and analogical perceptions are combined to reveal true insight.

When Fritz saw J.R. Worsley examine a patient and then talk about them, he asked himself, 'Where is he getting his information from?' The insights did not come from simply what they had said was happening and appeared to have a level of perception that was remarkable.

Ted Kaptchuk, in the second edition of his book on Chinese medicine, *The Web that Has No Weaver* (2000), devoted a chapter, 'Chinese Medicine as an Art', to his first teacher, Dr Hong Yuan-bain. The doctor exhibited a remarkably insightful perception characterised by 'seeing the whole in every part'. He was able to understand what was happening within a patient in an insightful, almost intuitive, manner. However, anyone who has studied in order to clinically apply these skills knows it comes through years of clinical development. Ted called the method of his teacher 'Tong Shen Ming', 'Penetrating Divine Illumination'. Its perception goes straight through to the subtlest level of the person's condition, 'penetrating (the essence) of the myriad things, as if the wind had blown the clouds away'.

> I first learned about this kind of vision from Dr Hong, my first teacher, who would routinely gain his patient's confidence by casually bringing up details of their life that they had not even mentioned before! He just knew. His intuition had been refined in a crucible of experience that gave him capacities beyond what is ordinarily thought possible... Just from being and talking with Dr Hong, most patients encountered within themselves a depth of humanity deeper than the difficulty or tragedy of any illness. Authenticity and integrity were experienced. The Qi shifted. The Spirit was touched. (Kaptchuk 2000, p.289)

I am also reminded of what Sir Arthur Conan Doyle described in a recording regarding his fictional detective Sherlock Holmes:

> I was when I wrote it a young doctor and had been educated in a very severe and critical medical school of thought. Especially coming under the influence of Dr Bell of Edinburgh who had most remarkable powers of observation. He prided himself that when he looked at a patient he could tell not only their disease, but very often their occupation and place of residence. Reading some detective stories I was struck by the fact that their results

were obtained in nearly every case by chance. I thought I would try my hand at writing a story where the hero would treat crime as Dr Bell treated disease and where science would take the place of chance. The result was Sherlock Holmes. I learned that many schools of detection working in France, Egypt and China have admittedly founded their system upon Holmes. To many he seems to be a real person. (Sir Arthur Conan Doyle, recorded in 1930)

Although Holmes claimed his conclusions came from deductive power, they demanded levels of attentive observation that may have been deemed irrelevant in a straightforward analytical approach. He saw and considered the whole picture in order to arrive at an accurate conclusion.

During his acupuncture studies with J.R. Worsley, Fritz's existing scientific structural analytical training was being challenged and complemented by learning an analogical approach. This seminal time was when Zero Balancing was being developed, before it was taught.

The practice of Zero Balancing develops and combines both approaches without contradiction. The anatomical knowledge discovered through analytical dissection is complemented by an energetic dimension, listening to the energy of qi through touch. The practice benefits from cultivating openness to the world from a place of inner silence. You can perceive the relative world of qi and its absolute origins in the *shen* spirit manifesting in the human body.

The cultivation of these skills through practice develops sensitivity and humanity. In ancient China the development of the practitioner of medicine implicitly involved an accompanying inner cultivation. It was almost taken as a given that the education of a doctor involved an awakening of their human consciousness, not merely the accumulation of information or techniques. I realise that during training in Western medicine part of the 'initiation' of junior doctors was for them to go through a period of intensive practice. These days this 'overwork' contravenes health and safety standards, but historically, this 'rite of passage' would often be the test by which they would transcend the previous level of their abilities.

Zero Balancing sessions can range from pleasantly relaxing and therapeutically beneficial to being potentially transformative through skilfully touching the hidden roots of imbalance.

The perception of interaction of the local and distal is active. Sensitive awareness to the 'working signs' of response that can indicate the client's structure and energy are engaged.

Zero Balancing works with a person's individual structure and energy, activating a universal intrinsic regulation, allowing a reordering and balance. There is a deep remembering and a true repairing when structure and energy are offered the opportunity to balance in a functioning unity.

The client is internally active within what might appear to be just a passive state. A Zero Balancing session is a non-verbal conversation. The client's structure and energy is evaluated, which begins the working relationship. Fulcrums and vectors engage accurately where they are required. With these held in place, the client's structure and energy takes the opportunity that is offered, and responds without force or compulsion. The phrase 'putting in a clearer, stronger force field' is better understood as setting up the conditions whereby change occurs, rather than demanding change. The Zero Balancer trusts in the knowledge of structural energetics to return a person to what is already there. The experience of 'clearer, stronger fields' is an outcome of awareness that comes out of their receptivity to what is naturally inherent. The Zero Balancer sets up the possibility, holding the person, and gets out of the way to allow nature to do the work. From a place of inner quietude the power of life in which you are an active being becomes evident.

Zero Balancing reconnects you with the larger fields of heaven, earth and humanity, returning you to a natural state of being alive. In Chinese this is known as *ziran*, that which is naturally so:

Human beings emulate the earth,
The earth emulates the heavens,
The heavens emulate the Dao,
The Dao emulates what is spontaneously so.

(Daodejing, *Chapter 25*)

Different therapies, depending on the breadth and depth of their understanding, have the potential to address various levels of healing. True healing has the potential to address disease, disposition and destiny. All medicine has an interest in disease in whatever way it sees or treats it. A holistic therapy not only addresses sickness but also recognises the root disposition that may underlie the variety of complaints. To treat at this level is treating the root of the person's imbalance, serving their fundamental health so they are less likely to become ill. Destiny in Chinese is seen in the character *ming*, understood as 'that which heaven has blessed you with'. Healing at this level is not just preventative but also brings you 'back on track', with a fuller awareness of fulfilling your life. It is valuable for the therapist to know where all three levels of their approaches might touch and to be open to their potential.

J.R. Worsley wrote in the introduction to *Is Acupuncture for You?* (1973, p.3):

> A practitioner of traditional acupuncture must strive to see patients not just as they are at the time of examination but as they would be if they were whole and perfect in body, mind and spirit, with every possibility of their unique being realised.

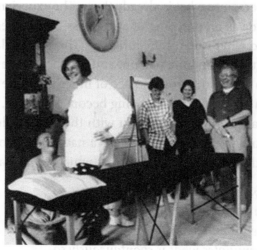

The joy of being Zero Balanced. Fritz Smith and students in a workshop

Appendix

The Influence of J.R. Worsley's Teaching in Dr Fritz Smith's Development of Zero Balancing

Professor J.R. Worsley and Dr Fritz Smith have both been pioneering teachers, inspiring generations of traditional acupuncturists and Zero Balancers to train, practise and, in turn, teach practitioners throughout Europe and North America. They proved their abilities in practice teaching, treating and touching thousands of people, demonstrating high-level skills. Fritz has often honoured J.R. Worsley as one of his key teachers, and acknowledged his importance in his own learning and discoveries about the structure and energy of our bodies and nature.

The experience for Fritz of studying with J.R. Worsley gave him working contact with a practitioner working with a structural energetic therapy of Oriental origin that intrinsically recognised body-mind-spirit. J.R. Worsley also showed that the skills and understanding involved in their practice were accessible and could be inspirationally taught to and practised by others. He brought an ancient theoretical and practical knowledge vividly alive, and proved its power and contemporary clinical relevance. This unlocked the doorway to what might appear an esoteric, hidden mystery, and bridged the worlds of ancient and modern, East and West.

Fritz first met J.R. Worsley in 1971 when he taught a seminar on traditional acupuncture at the Esalen Institute in California. Fritz was encouraged to attend this event by his wife Betty and by the systems biologist Gregory Bateson, renowned author of *Mind and Nature* (1979). Fritz had successfully treated Gregory Bateson's wife and he recommended Fritz attend this event. It turned out to be seminal. The experience of seeing J.R. Worsley treat is described vividly in Fritz's book *Inner Bridges* (1986, p.182): 'As I listened to this treatment report my mind seemed to explode; none of my medical experience could account for what I was hearing. It was shortly after that I committed myself to the study of energy and our subtle nature.'

J.R. Worsley would talk about a patient after he had examined them in ways that were deeply insightful. Fritz has said he was not initially so interested in studying acupuncture as finding out 'Where is he getting his information from?' Fritz was also inspired by encountering a practitioner who was treating using an anatomy of the structure and energy of the body that fundamentally challenged the existing knowledge he knew, learned through his osteopathic and medical studies. The patient J.R. Worsley treated presented with a constriction of one hand which, after ten years, had not responded to any other investigative or treatment intervention: 'I learned that only a single point had been used and this had been placed in the soft tissue of the opposite leg. The needle was kept in place for about ten seconds.' The patient 'walked out of the consultation room, closing his hand fully for the first time in ten years. He was ecstatic.'

Fritz witnessed this demonstration of the effectiveness of acupuncture around the time that it was very much in the news. *The New York Times* reporter James Reston had written of his experience of having acupuncture when he went to China, reporting on Nixon's visit to Mao in 1972. This had been followed by lively discussions that Fritz attended at Stanford about the efficacy of acupuncture.

From Fritz's accounts of his initial meeting with J.R. Worsley at the Esalen Institute, it appears that they both 'hit it off' from the start. They sensed an instinctive empathy of two explorers in the same field who had much to learn and share together, a genuine meeting of body-mind-spirits. They may have come from different backgrounds, but they felt an essential connection of being on a common path.

Fritz travelled to England with a group of Americans to study acupuncture and continued his studies, completing a Master's in Acupuncture degree and clinical observation and continuing contact with J.R. Worsley until his death. The training in 1972 was organised by Bob Duggan and Dianne Connelly, who, on returning to the USA, founded the Traditional Acupuncture Institute (TAI) in Maryland with their fellow students. Fritz was a major supporter of TAI and regularly taught Zero Balancing to acupuncture students, spoke at its conferences and contributed articles to its journal, *Meridians*.

It has been frequently noted that Fritz began to formulate the development of Zero Balancing when he wrote about it as his project of excellence for his Bachelor's degree. He was also encouraged to recognise that Zero Balancing could be taught to others by an English student who attended the same acupuncture course, Julia Measures. She told Fritz of the very positive responses from those she had touched, using what she had learnt from Fritz. This enthused him and confirmed the idea that this was a practical approach that could be effectively shared with others. Fritz's fellow American student on the course, Jim McCormick, also began to share Zero Balancing with others, which stimulated Fritz into structuring Zero Balancing into an 'information-sharing workshop' presentation for healthcare practitioners.

J.R. Worsley was clear that the skills he was using required the development of a full range of sensory awareness, interacting with a patient to see, hear, smell and touch the state of their qi. This information gave direct insight into the interior state of functioning and balance of a person's qi, observable at a body level. For example, the colour of their internal qi is visible and embodied on their face, not in some 'auric field' or in a hidden level. The basis of these skills has been recorded by the Chinese in the *Yellow Emperor's Inner Classic* as a key aspect of classical medicine from the third century BC. At the time Fritz began his studies, the only English translation of this major text was a partial one by an American academic, Ilza Veith. J.R. Worsley was adamant that you couldn't learn acupuncture from books. Indeed, they would fill you up with ideas that could impede your practical development. Both J.R. Worsley and Fritz recognised that in order to sense the person's qi, you had to get 'out of your head' and into your senses in ways that transcended the education a Westerner usually brings to try and understand the world. J.R. Worsley was teaching a discipline that had objectivity and was not merely personal subjective projection or judgement. The skill requires you to quieten the mind, awaken your attention and know or recognise yourself so that you transcend any personal bias that might influence your perceptions. This objectivity demanded sensitivity to the structure and energy of the patient's qi and to know where the person ended and you began for clarity. Whilst J.R. Worsley did not come from a meditative tradition, he clearly brought a particular internal discipline and rigour to his clinical skills. This developed a complementary approach to the way the West usually analysed information and judged, with a tendency to a tunnel vision conclusion. It involved a sensory acuity, becoming aware of the wider picture and gathering information in the context of the larger picture. This skill is also known in the West in the term *gestalt*, where your perceptions require you to see both figure and ground, inner and outer, structure and energy, as an interactive whole. It also brings an insight into what, within any circumstance, is incongruent with the whole – for example, in traditional acupuncture, a colour or pulse not matching with other information gathered.

J.R. Worsley developed his senses and diagnostic insight in ways which, to anyone not aware of the tradition he was drawing on, might appear 'intuitive' or extraordinary. He then used the refinement of his perception to craft simple but fundamental acupuncture treatments, through which he furthered the knowledge he gained of the patient. He was alive to their responsiveness to treatment and the level of their condition, monitoring them throughout the session using pulse, colour, sound, emotion and odour. This attention to these 'working signs' of patient response and knowing when enough treatment was complete for that session inspired Fritz to gather these observations into his practice and teaching of Zero Balancing.

Fritz brought the awareness of touch and evaluating the body's structure and energy from his own education and development to complement the sensory skills J.R. Worsley was teaching. J.R. Worsley was very hands-on in his clinical examination of patients, a fact often lost by later teachers of his approach. J.R. Worsley would touch the patient's body with a gentle yet firm manner to engage their structure and qi. This was evident in his pulse taking, feeling the temperature of the patient's trunk (Three Jiao), feeling the pathways on their limbs and head pathways, touching for spontaneous tenderness at known points (Mu 'alarm points'), finding the umbilical pulse and abdominal palpation (*hara*). He had had training in physiotherapy in the Second World War and after the war was exposed to other students of acupuncture who came from an osteopathic background, who then introduced him to the art of osteopathic manipulation.

J.R. Worsley's pulse taking was practised standing, with the patient lying comfortably on their back. It involved the practitioner holding the hand of the patient with their opposite hand and palpating their radial pulse with the fingers of their other hand, one at a time, at two different depths, reading the relative quantity and quality of different pulses on both wrists. This is quite different from how pulses are usually taken in China, where the practitioner sits beside the patient who rests their wrist on a small cushion on a ZB table.

J.R. Worsley had also brilliantly demonstrated how to bring your attention to the patient being examined, and then treating them in ways that engaged them, developing the kind of rapport and trust we know occurs in Zero Balancing. He would carefully monitor their response to needling each point through observation of pulse change and other levels of sensing change in the patient. Many acupuncturists put needles in and sit back reading a book, or even leaving the patient in the treatment room. Some practitioners treat without even feeling the pulse. The attention to monitoring changes in the patient was developed by Fritz in his 'working signs' of changes in a person when they are undergoing a therapy that touches their energy. Fritz said he was struck by observing J.R. Worsley go from room to room when he was instructing practitioners who were treating patients and opening a door, glancing at a patient and saying 'the treatment is complete'. Working signs also incorporate observation of the practice of other modalities, but are clearly inspired by observing J.R. Worsley's mastery in the treatment room.

The particular and relatively unusual way J.R. Worsley used needles is often not fully recognised. His technique probably derived from more Japanese approaches, and is quite distinct from the more 'physical' Chinese methods that are commonly practised. J.R. Worsley's needling has been described as 'butterfly'-like. It had a subtle power whereby the patient might not even be aware of much sensation or the *de qi* (obtaining qi), the cramping ache that is usually a requirement of Chinese needling. Yet the patient's response was palpable on the pulse and observable in their colour, sound, odour and emotion. J.R. Worsley used relatively thin gauge needles, very different to contemporary practice that often favours considerably thicker needles where the patient is all too aware of having something done to them. Zero Balancing often works beneath the client's full level of awareness, until they get up off the ZB table. It also follows a rhythm of evaluation, introducing fulcrums and vectors that work with the person, and then re-evaluating, to sensitively guide and pace the Zero Balancing. A session does not overload with more fulcrums than are needed, but is tailored to match their structural energetic needs. It similarly develops a practice that works with the patient rather than doing something to them.

Another characteristic of J.R. Worsley's treatments was that he used needles relatively sparingly compared with some acupuncturists who might use many more needles in one session. Having examined and diagnosed a patient, he would select only a few points. A patient might get just two points, needled bilaterally, in a single treatment. These would often be selected distally from the site of the person's complaint. This was based on a clear understanding of the state and balance of their elements, organ officials and meridian pathways, with a highly developed awareness of the value and spirit of each point. This approach addressed the underlying roots of the patient's condition with a keen awareness of what, in Zero Balancing, we know as 'the other end of the string' of interacting local–distal relationships.

J.R. Worsley's approach also anchored and grounded a treatment using fundamental points located on the lower limbs of the arms and hands, which are known as points that fundamentally command the balance and quality of the qi. If he needled a point on the trunk or head he would complement it with points on the arms or legs to relate this to the patient's underlying root needs, and integrate local with distal structure and energy. He also commonly combined needling both yin and yang, inner and outer pairings of pathways related to a specific element. This is not in any way a common practice in acupuncture, but reflects a way of keeping a fundamental balance within an element. This can be seen in Zero Balancing by Fritz emphasising that any local work, for example on freely moveable joints or one sided on the body, is integrated by vectors or fulcrums that allow this work to be recognised by the rest of the patient's body and become a whole body experience.

In Chinese medicine terms J.R. Worsley diagnosed and treated the roots of a patient's condition rather than the branches. A fundamental appreciation of classical treatment is to discern and address the underlying root of the pathologies which the person may be complaining about, rather than palliate the 'branches' of their symptomatology. In Zero Balancing this can be seen as the way core Zero Balancing pays attention to the foundation and semi-foundation joints. States of imbalance in these are often beneath a person's normal awareness or ability to alter or rebalance, and yet can have widespread ramifications for their health. Zero Balancing also has the awareness that an imbalance in a person's body may reflect distally at other places far away from the site of the imbalanced joint and also in the way they experience themselves in other ways than physical, for example in mood, manner or outlook. Balancing these fundamental joints in themselves and in coherent relationship with others elsewhere in the patient's body is a focus of core Zero Balancing. Both J.R. Worsley and Fritz's teachings therefore feature as an approach that perceives and addresses the fundamentals of a person's structure and energy in their own ways, and teachers regard this as core.

J.R. Worsley's treatments could often be transformational for the patient. This reflected the way that treatments are at a root level, with awareness of the way points can touch a person in the subtle power of their spirits and their qi energy. J.R. Worsley characterised the points and brought their nature and power alive by describing their 'spirit', and was aware of how a point could affect both their structural functioning as well as their emotional wellbeing. He was conscious that, as Jung said, much of the disease of modern man came from a separation from Nature and his inner nature. Both J.R. Worsley and Fritz have often said that, to understand the structure and energy or the condition of a person, 'look to nature' for examples and insights.

J.R. Worsley's teaching had an immediate appeal to those seeking knowledge, perfectly timed in the growing ecological awareness of the second half of the twentieth century and the expansion of awareness through the 1960s. His teaching was characterised by easily understood analogies in the way qi exhibits in the element nature, for example Fire, Water, Wood, Metal and Earth, and in the way these manifest viscerally as officials. This latter insight (drawing on *The Yellow Emperor's Inner Classic*, *Su Wen*, Chapter 8) brought their functioning alive as a working bureaucracy within us, under the leadership of the Heart. The brilliance of this anthropomorphic teaching allows an ancient knowledge of the body-mind-spirit to be immediately understood by the practitioner in an everyday way they could relate to and grasp. This should be seen in the context of so-called 'Traditional Chinese Medicine' of the post-revolutionary medicine in modern China where the organs (in Chinese, *Zang-fu*) were seen and treated in a more 'physical' level of functioning to bring them in line with contemporary biomedicine, in a move to bring this knowledge in line with Western medical practice. One of the characteristics of Zero Balancing is to make its practice and knowledge comprehensible to the everyday person as well – not esoteric or unnecessarily intellectual, but well anchored in information that allows the mind to comprehend it. Learning is accompanied by hands-on practice so that it becomes an embodied education. A student understands this information through engaging the body's structure and energy rather than trying to figure it out with their intellect and then attempting to put this into practice – understanding it directly in your hands rather than only intellectually. This in no way means a denial of our intelligence, but is a way of learning that can help transcend the separation of mind and body. It is so often lacking in Western education where somebody's apparent knowledge of the concepts and ideas is dislocated from their ability to demonstrate these in practice.

The ways J.R. Worsley and Fritz taught both acupuncture and Zero Balancing respectively share a common characteristic of simplicity of fundamental theory that is enjoyably and accessibly grasped. Many other approaches may appear to have more 'information' but often disguise their weaknesses with a thicket of concepts and ideas, turning education into an information overload of academic respectability, where an ongoing struggle between brain and body eclipses the spirit of the original teaching, or reduces it to a mere intellectual belief system.

Zero Balancing touches a person at the level of their core structure, their bones, whilst simultaneously touching their energy. Therefore the most solid, palpable tissue of their form is contacted at the same time as the subtle life of their qi and spirits. In his needling J.R. Worsley was aware that it was not some mechanical insertion of metal into physical tissue, but involved sensitively entering the body with care, attention and respect to engage the structure and qi of the living body. In acupuncture this is qi that is accessible within the connective tissues. In Zero Balancing, the structure and energy is engaged at the level of bone.

What is remarkable is J.R. Worsley's way of needling. A large number of acupuncturists insert needles that are then left in (retained), whether they are tonifying or dispersing. J.R. Worsley's most frequent use of needles for tonification involved needles being inserted, manipulated and then removed without retention within a few seconds. The patient's pulse would be felt to monitor the treatment and to decide whether more points were required. The unusual nature of his needling is not frequently recognised. In Zero Balancing, fulcrums and vectors are introduced, held for a few seconds, and then released. There may be a pause, followed by re-evaluation, and then moving on to another joint or area of the body. The rhythm of this process of evaluation, fulcrum and re-evaluation with frequent disconnection is often distinct from many bodywork approaches, for example massage, where you may be encouraged to be in constant contact with a person throughout the session, or the Bowen technique, where practitioners may even leave the room following a procedure for a while before returning. Zero Balancing is like an interactive dance, frequently similar to the manner J.R. Worsley conducted a treatment. The practitioner's attention and involvement is present throughout the session. There is an engagement and awareness of how the patient responds, and integrating the treatment so they fully assimilate its benefits.

The other important aspect of J.R. Worsley's needling in relation to Zero Balancing is the apparent simplicity of his needle technique. J.R. Worsley would insert the needle to the depth and then rotate it 180 degrees (for tonification) and then remove it. In Zero Balancing the body's structure and energy is engaged with the appreciation of what is known as the 'blue line'. A fulcrum is held for a few seconds and then released. A fulcrum works best when the person's structure and energy are properly engaged. A fulcrum can be a simple lifting, but the relationship with structure and energy is often best built on by simply compounding it with another plane, such as turning it 180 degrees. The effectiveness of this way of engaging and working with the structure and energy of the body has been affirmed in independent studies.

A fundamental aspect of J.R. Worsley's approach to healing with acupuncture was to harmonise the relationships between the elements and officials through ways of fundamental balancing. This was often accomplished through 'transfers' between the elements and officials, harmonising their relationships through treatments utilising the *sheng* and *ko* cycle of their interrelationships that rule their inner generation and control. This classical approach is quite distinct from diagnosing a symptom and the treatment of syndromes seen in post-revolutionary 'Traditional Chinese Medicine'.

J.R. Worsley treated people as unique individuals rather than labelling them as pathologies. He addressed the underlying im-balance rather than treating or palliating their symptoms. He was interested in the underlying roots that had led to their health declining and their becoming ill. He also followed the classic dictum that you don't start digging a well when you become thirsty, meaning that the proper way of treating a person is before they become in anyway ill or in decline. He treated in ways that tuned a person to the rhythms of nature as they negotiated changes in life. This classical use of acupuncture is also the approach followed in Zero Balancing. It is not being used as a 'fix it' therapy but more as a way of clearing and harmonising the underlying field of the patient's qi energy. It is also excellent in returning a person to themselves, keeping them on track in their life, and enabling them to respond to the stresses in life through a flexible transmission in their structure and energy that enables adaptability to change and enlivens homeostasis. This is truly preventative medicine praised by the ancient Chinese as well as by modern healthcare.

Both teachers recognised that the disciplines they taught implicitly demanded continuing education to grow and deepen the nature of their skills. Both disciplines could be described as being an ongoing path of learning. Both can be named as true practice that nurtures the practitioners who work with them if they recognise the development of awareness required in their activity. This was well before any Continuing Professional Development requirement was made by an external body. It was taken as an obvious given, inherent to anyone who grasped its nature. Both teachers showed an unending curiosity through their practice, an interest in continued learning and 'growing edge' of discovery that had originally attracted them. Traditional acupuncture and Zero Balancing both have the possibility of cultivating the authentic nature of those who practise them.

Fritz's time of studying with J.R. Worsley in the 1970s gave him the opportunity to reflect on the nature of his previous education as well as his training with Ida Rolf and other formative experiences. It allowed him to appreciate the knowledge of anatomy and the body's functioning he had gained through osteopathy, and to see it in relation to the wider context of the energy medicine of acupuncture. The requirements of writing up a project of excellence paper for his Bachelor in Acupuncture degree gave him the opportunity to formalise the ferment of his insights. The environment of being with receptive and supportive fellow students encouraged him, confirming that this was a worthwhile approach that had significant therapeutic benefits which both complemented what he was learning with J.R. Worsley and could also stand as a therapy in its own right.

Selected Bibliography

Al-Khalili, J. and McFadden, J. (2014) *Life on the Edge: The Coming of Age of Quantum Biology*. London: Bantam Press.

Ames, R.T. and Hall, D.L. (2003) *Dao De Jing*. New York: Ballantine Books.

Bateson, G. (1979) *Mind and Nature*. New York: E.P. Dutton.

Becker, R.O. and Selden, G. (1985) *The Body Electric: Electromagnetism and the Foundation of Life*. New York: William Morrow.

Birch, S., Mir, M.A.C. and Cuadras, M.R. (2014) *Restoring Order in Health and Chinese Medicine*. Barcelona: La Liebre de Marzo.

Bromley, M., Freeman, D., Hext, A. and Hill, S., under the aegis of E. Rochat de la Vallée (2010) *Jing Shen: A Translation of Huainanzi Chapter 7*. London: Monkey Press.

Calais-Germain, B. (1993) *Anatomy of Movement*. Seattle, WA: Eastland Press.

Capra, F. and Luisi, P.L. (2014) *The Systems View of Life: A Unifying Vision*. Cambridge: Cambridge University Press.

Chung-Yuan, C. (1963) *Creativity and Taoism*. New York: Harper & Row Publishers.

Dürckheim, K.G. (1962) *Hara: The Vital Centre of Man*. London: George Allen & Unwin.

Ellis, A., Wiseman, N. and Boss, K. (1989) *Grasping the Wind*. Brookline, MA: Paradigm Publications.

Feitis, R. (ed.) (1978) *Ida Rolf Talks about Rolfing and Physical Reality*. St Paul, MN: Bookslinger.

Foster, R.G. and Kreitzman, L. (2017) *Circadian Rhythms*. Oxford: Oxford University Press.

Fung, Y.-L. (1953) *A History of Chinese Philosophy, Volume II*. Princeton, NJ: Princeton University Press.

Gardner, M. (1964) *The Ambidextrous Universe*. Harmondsworth: Pelican – Penguin.

Gorman, D. (1981) *The Body Moveable*. Ontario, Canada: Ampersand Press.

Hamwee, J. (1999) *Zero Balancing*. London: Frances Lincoln.

Hartley, L. (1989) *Wisdom of the Body Moving: An Introduction to Body-Mind Centering*. Berkeley, CA: North Atlantic Books.

Ho, M.-W. (1998) *The Rainbow and the Worm: The Physics of Organisms*. Singapore: World Scientific Publishing.

Ichazo, O. (1986) *Master Level Exercise: Psychocalisthenics*. Bellevue, WA: Sequoia Press.

Kapandji, I.A. (1974) *The Physiology of Joints: In Three Volumes*. Edinburgh: Churchill Livingstone.

Kaplan, R. (1999) *The Nothing that Is: A Natural History of Zero*. Harmondsworth: Allen Lane, Penguin Press.

Kaptchuk, T. (2000) *The Web that Has No Weaver*, 2nd edn. Chicago, IL: Contemporary Publishing Group.

Koestler, A. (1975) *The Act of Creation*. London: Picador.

Larre, C. and Rochat de la Vallée, E. (1997) *The Eight Extraordinary Meridians*. London: Monkey Press.

Larre, C., Schatz, J. and Rochat de la Vallée, E. (1986) *Survey of Traditional Chinese Medicine*. Columbia, MD: Traditional Acupuncture Foundation and the Ricci Institute.

Lauterstein, D. (2011) *The Deep Massage Book: How to Combine Structure and Energy in Bodywork*. Taos, NM: Complementary Medicine Press.

Lauterstein, D. (2017) *Life in the Bones: A Biography of Dr Fritz Smith and Zero Balancing*. Palm Beach Gardens, FL: Upledger Productions.

Legge, J. (1971) *Confucius: Analects, The Great Learning and The Doctrine of the Mean*. New York: Dover Publications.

Man-ch'ing, C. (1997) *Essays on Man and Culture*. Palo Alto, CA: Frog Ltd.

Needham, J. (1962) *Science and Civilisation in China*. Volume 2. Cambridge: Cambridge University Press.

Oschman, J. (2000) *Energy Medicine: The Scientific Basis*. Edinburgh: Churchill Livingstone.

Oschman, J. (2003) *Energy Medicine in Therapeutics and Human Performance*. Edinburgh: Butterworth and Heinemann.

Quarry, V. and King, A. (2016) *Experiencing the Power of Zero Balancing*. Palm Beach Gardens, FL: Upledger Productions.

Rochat de la Vallée, E. (1999) *Essence, Spirit, Blood and Qi*. London: Monkey Press.

Rochat de la Vallée, E. (2006) *A Study of Qi*. London: Monkey Press.

Rochat de la Vallée, E. (2006) *Yin Yang*. London: Monkey Press.

Rochat de la Vallée, E. (2009) *Wu Xing: The Five Elements*. London: Monkey Press.

Rochat de la Vallée, E. (2011) *The Rhythm at the Heart of the World: Neijing Suwen Chapter 5*. London: Monkey Press.

Shrödinger, E. (1967) *What is Life? With Mind and Matter*. Cambridge: Cambridge University Press.

Smith, F.F. (1986) *Inner Bridges: A Guide to Energy Movement and Body Structure*. Atlanta, GA: Humanics Ltd.

Smith, F.F. (2005) *The Alchemy of Touch: Moving towards Mastery through the Lens of Zero Balancing*. Taos, NM: Complementary Medicine Press.

Soeng, M. (2010) *The Heart of the Universe: Exploring the Heart Sutra*. Boston, MA: Wisdom Publications.

Stiskin, M.N. (1971) *The Looking Glass God*. Tokyo: Autumn Press.

Sullivan, J. (2014) *Zero Balancing Expanded*. Palm Beach Gardens, FL: Upledger Productions.

Suzuki, S. (1970) *Zen Mind, Beginner's Mind*. New York: Weatherhill.

Thompson, D'A. (1961) *On Growth and Form*. Cambridge: Cambridge University Press.

Watson, B. (1968) *The Complete Works of Chuang Tzu*. New York: Columbia University Press.

Watts, A. (1963) *The Two Hands of God: The Myths of Polarity*. New York: Macmillan.

Watts, A. (1974) *Cloud Hidden, Whereabouts Unknown*. New York: Vintage Books.

Worsley, J.R. (1973) *Is Acupuncture for You?* New York: Harper & Row.

Worsley, J.R. (1982) *Traditional Chinese Acupuncture Vol. 1: Meridians and Points*. Tisbury: Element Books.

Worsley, J.R. (1998) *The Five Elements and the Officials*. London: J.R. and J.B. Worsley.

Yoke, H.P. (1985) *Li, Qi and Shu: An Introduction to Science and Civilization in China*. Hong Kong: Hong Kong University Press.

Index